Understanding AIDS

Understanding AIDS

Dr John Starkie and Rodney Dale

Published by
Consumers' Association
and Hodder & Stoughton

Which? Books are commissioned by The Association for Consumer
Research and published by Consumers' Association, 2 Marylebone
Road, London NW1 4DX and Hodder & Stoughton Ltd,
47 Bedford Square, London WC1B 3DP

British Library Cataloguing in Publication Data

Starkie, John
Understanding AIDS.
1. Man. AIDS
I. Title II. Dale, Rodney, 1933–
III. Consumers' Association
616.9'792

ISBN 0 340 41621 1

Cover illustration: John Holder
Typesetting: Goodfellow & Egan Ltd, Cambridge
Design and artwork: Business Literature Services Ltd, Cambridge
Printed and bound in Great Britain by Hazell Watson & Viney Ltd
Member of the BPCC plc
Aylesbury, Bucks

CONTENTS

AUTHORS' ACKNOWLEDGEMENTS

We would like to thank many helpful librarians, particularly at the Clinical School in the University of Cambridge, and at the Royal Society of Medicine. We thank also our wives, Judith Dale, who scoured the press for AIDS material, and Margaret Starkie, who acted as midwife to the draft copy.

We are grateful to Julia Beavis, Katie Bent and Christine Pawley, who worked shifts to decipher and word-process our manuscripts; Christine also prepared the discs for typesetting. We owe a particular debt of gratitude to Trish Morris, who contributed indefatigably by managing the project and retaining a sense of humour through a daunting sequence of tasks. Our thanks also to Rob Attwood who prepared the diagrams and artwork. The caption to the diagram of the lymph system, on page 41, is based on explanations in Consumers' Association's book, *Understanding Cancer*.

Whatever imperfections remain must be laid at our doors.

INTRODUCTION

This book was born in 1986 when people were starting to worry about a new and deadly disease. At that time, few of us knew very much about it. Now AIDS has become a topic of everyday conversation. Information pours from the government, the media, school and church, friends and family. Yet somehow it seems that the plethora of information makes the subject even more confusing – worse, there is a danger that those at risk are becoming blasé. So the book that started as a source of information is even more important now than it was then.

Our purpose is to present the facts; to dispel the mystery; to explain what AIDS is and how it might affect us, our families, our friends and acquaintances – and to determine exactly how worried we should be. Is this the beginning of the end of the world or – to go to the other extreme – is AIDS something nasty which affects certain minority groups and which will go away in its own time?

As we found out more about AIDS we realised what a difficult subject it is; it touches on matters which many people find unpalatable, and there is an admixture of myth and truth. We believe that the rapidly-changing perceptions stem chiefly from one cause – a lack of understanding. Hence the title of this book *Understanding AIDS*; an understanding of a subject will enable anyone to judge the wisdom or otherwise of various courses of action; the dangers inherent in them; the truth or falsity of statements made.

Suddenly, as we started to write this book, AIDS was in the news every single day – the public was bombarded with AIDS – in the newspapers and magazines, on television, at the cinema, on the streets – and it was an inevitable topic of conversation. It was impossible not to absorb something about AIDS. For some there was too much about AIDS – overkill. People were bored with hearing about AIDS. 'We know all about AIDS,' they would say, or: 'AIDS is deadly – but it's not likely to happen to anyone I know, certainly not me.'

By February 1988, 1,344 people in the UK were reported as having had AIDS – 749 of them had died. The number of cases doubles every year. By January 1988 there were 8,016 diagnosed cases of HIV infection in the UK.

As our task neared its end, the reality of AIDS was beginning to strike; many people now knew – or knew someone who knew – someone with AIDS. We saw that it was even more important for the message to be universally received; our main concern is that those who do not read it – or heed it – may also be those most at risk. Hence again the importance of understanding, and passing on that understanding to others.

What we have done is to sift through the research of many scientists, and the mass of information more accessible to the public, in order to provide a clear view which rules out the contradictions and misconceptions arising from the interpretations of lobby groups and the media.

We have presented this in such a way that readers can relate AIDS to their own lifestyles – and those of their families and friends. We would like to dispel the unnecessary fears of some and instil more concern in others who have got so bored with the subject that they no longer care.

Above all, we want to promote understanding of AIDS – a disease which has become an integral part of today's society, and which remains, as yet, incurable.

John Starkie
Rodney Dale

1   What AIDS is – and isn't

AIDS

AIDS is a disease that results from infection with a virus called Human Immunodeficiency Virus (HIV), which spreads from person to person in body fluids.

In its early stages the virus causes an illness, which we have called the primary illness, sometimes similar to glandular fever. The primary illness may not be obvious, as it may come and go, but eventually it destroys the body's resistance to infections and cancers.

AIDS develops later, is debilitating and usually fatal. During the course of the disease the patient has several infections, or cancers, or a combination of both. In healthy people, such infections and cancers are rejected by the body, and so may pass unnoticed, but in an AIDS patient they cause serious illness and are eventually fatal.

HIV

The Human Immunodeficiency Virus is a relatively new virus, and may have infected human beings for only twenty years or so. It is spread from person to person in body fluids, such as blood, seminal fluid and vaginal mucus, but is probably not spread by droplets from coughing and sneezing, and is certainly not spread by touching.

In Chapter 2 we describe the groups of people that are most likely to have HIV and those people most likely to catch it. Those who, because of their lifestyle, are most likely to have the virus, or to catch it, are said to belong to a *high-risk group*. 'Risk' is a statistical concept, and can be given a value: the higher the value, the greater the risk. Statisticians refer to groups, such as 'homosexual men', 'drug addicts', 'heterosexuals', 'lesbians' and so on. People in some groups are more likely to have, or to catch, HIV than people in other groups; we have listed our four examples in decreasing order of risk. Within each group of people the risk is not the same for each person; some individuals in a group are more likely to have or to catch HIV than others in the same group.

Because of this variability, many stories have arisen about who can catch HIV, how it is spread, and how people can avoid getting AIDS. Chapter 3 quotes some of these stories and tries to comment simply on whether they are true or false. In some cases not enough is known to give a simple 'yes' or 'no'; in such cases we have described what is known.

HIV is a new, and slightly different, form of a virus that scientists have studied for some years. Similar viruses cause feline leukaemia (in cats only), others cause a kind of leukaemia, and other blood cancers, in people, yet other forms of the virus cause a kind of AIDS in some monkeys. We explain how HIV works in Chapter 4.

The Syndrome

The primary illness of HIV usually leads on to AIDS. The initials AIDS stand for Acquired Immune Deficiency Syndrome. A syndrome is a collection of signs and symptoms, such as loss of weight, swelling of glands, diarrhoea. We describe more fully the signs and symptoms that are characteristic of AIDS in Chapter 5.

Immune deficiency (immunodeficiency) is a state in which a person's resistance (immunity) to infection is reduced. Chapters 4 and 5 explain how HIV infects the cells that protect the body against infections and cancers. In Chapter 5 we list and describe some of the infections and cancers that result from the immune deficiency of AIDS, and which cause the deaths of people with AIDS. These infections are described as opportunistic because they grasp the opportunity offered them by their victims' lowered resistance.

AIDS results from an infection with HIV, which in turn is spread by the transfer of infected body fluid from an infected person to a non-infected person. The body fluids most usually implicated in the spread of HIV from person to person are blood and seminal fluid. Chapter 6 deals specifically with blood and Chapter 7 shows how we know that there are other body fluids which spread HIV, and describes in some detail how HIV, and therefore AIDS, is spread from person to person. The chapter links the risk of catching HIV — and AIDS — with the lifestyles which people have adopted, and with the groups into which statisticians have placed people. It also shows how the risk for an individual within a group of people might be quite different from the risk for the group as a whole. For example, the risk for lesbian women — as a group — is quite low, but the risk for a lesbian woman who chose to become pregnant by means of artificial insemination with semen from a Californian homosexual man would be very high — as was proved in the mid-1980s (see Chapter 7).

The emergence of AIDS

AIDS was first recorded in a group of Californian homosexual men in 1979: before then it was unknown. However, by 1987 people had died of AIDS in every country in the world. Chapter 8 describes how HIV might have originated in central Africa, and how it might have spread to the Caribbean and to the US cities of Los Angeles, San Francisco and New York. It is clear that from there, and from central Africa, the virus spread rapidly to the rest of the developed world, and then back to Africa and the rest of the developing world.

For those who think they might have become infected with HIV, there are clinical tests. At the time of writing (Spring 1988) the tests may still not be easily available. Although for the person being tested they simply require taking a sample of blood, they are technically complex, and therefore expensive. Chapter 9 describes the tests and the clinical implications of the results. It also discusses some of the social and financial implications of being tested and of the result. It goes on to suggest how those with the virus can avoid transmitting it to other people. The overriding principle is to avoid passing infected body fluid into another person's body.

A cure for AIDS?

People who become infected have the hope of a cure within the next ten years. A vaccine might protect uninfected people from becoming infected, but is not likely to prevent AIDS developing if HIV is already in the bloodstream. Moreover, a vaccine for HIV is more difficult to prepare than a vaccine against, say, polio or smallpox, as we explain in Chapter 10. The best hope for 1988 and 1989 is that one of the anti-viral drugs being tested will be effective, and will not have dangerous side-effects.

For people infected with HIV, and for people with AIDS, the prime aim must be to stay as healthy as possible — both mentally and physically – for as long as possible. There are several mutual help schemes to provide comfort, friendship and hope. There are diets and fitness regimes that claim to delay the effects of infections, and hospices specifically for people in the terminal stages of AIDS are beginning to open. Chapter 11 considers how a person with AIDS, and their friends, should try to cope with the illness. Chapter 12 lists organisations in England, Scotland and Wales that offer information, advice and counselling on all aspects of AIDS; many of them operate telephone helplines.

AIDS is a venereal disease (that is, transmitted by sexual intercourse) but can be transmitted in other ways. As a result, some people have seen AIDS as retribution on the permissive and promiscuous; others have warned that it is a danger to the survival of mankind. From a scientific point of view, HIV is a virus that mutated at a time when the lifestyles of very many people in the developed world changed quite markedly, and which, as a result, has become prevalent across the world – pandemic.

There is no doubt that measures will be found to prevent the spread of AIDS; cures will be found which will be more or less effective. But these discoveries will take time, and during that time a lot of people will die of AIDS. But even when prevention and cure become possible some people will ignore both, just as some people now ignore the prevention and cure of syphilis and whooping cough. If AIDS were not venereal, it might be possible to eliminate the virus from the world, like smallpox. But because HIV is transmitted by sexual intercourse and because it has a long incubation time, it is likely that a residue of AIDS will remain in all permissive societies.

Comparisons with other diseases

AIDS can be compared with a number of other diseases, but often the only link is that both are caused by a virus and both are fatal.

Smallpox

Both smallpox and AIDS are caused by a virus. Not so long ago, smallpox was feared in much the same way that AIDS is now. However, the two viruses are very different.

Although, unlike AIDS, smallpox did not always result in death, survivors were usually severely pockmarked and disfigured for life, often on the face, where disfigurement is most obvious.

Smallpox was feared by everyone: no one thought that there might be a lifestyle which would prevent their catching smallpox. It was more immediate and obvious to the public eye than is AIDS. The HIV epidemic is virtually unseen, as symptoms of AIDS may not appear for two years or more after infection and no one can tell who is infected, not even the victims. Smallpox, on the other hand, had an incubation period of not more than 16 days. Cause and effect were close in time and obvious in relationship.

Another difference between AIDS and smallpox is the method of spread from person to person. The smallpox virus was spread by droplet infection from the lungs and throat, during coughing and sneezing and by contamination with the fluid from the pocks. Smallpox was contagious: it could be caught by being in the same room, or even the same street, as an infected person. HIV, on the other hand, is transmitted only by an exchange of body fluids. The virus does not survive in droplets in the air, and is not contagious.

Paradoxically, this major difference tends to make AIDS *more* feared than smallpox. Avoiding a smallpox patient was fairly easy, especially after the incubation period: news of a victim travelled faster than the virus.

AIDS is different. For some people exchange of body fluids is difficult to control or avoid. Haemophiliacs may die if they don't infuse Factor VIII; accident victims have little choice about receiving blood transfusions. Also, the sexual urge is so strong, instinctive and nowadays acceptable, that it may be difficult to control the transfer of saliva, vaginal fluid and seminal fluid. This, coupled with the very long incubation period, makes for a less rapid, but more thorough, spread of AIDS.

Another vital difference between smallpox and AIDS is that some people seemed to be immune to smallpox — they never became infected. Others recovered from the disease and were able to nurse yet others, without fear of a second infection. It was subsequently shown that infection with the cowpox virus conferred immunity against smallpox without traces of disease — indeed, this is how the principle of vaccination was discovered.

Little is known for certain about immunity from AIDS. It has not been established whether transfer of infected body fluid *always* results in infection; there is equally no evidence to the contrary. There is no evidence that anyone becomes immune to the virus, although it might happen. Not everyone who is infected with HIV has developed AIDS, even after eight years (since records were kept), but it is widely believed by experts that the disease is inevitable after infection.

Smallpox can now be prevented by vaccination, and the World Health Organisation claims that it has been eradicated from the world. However, the nature of HIV makes it more difficult to find a vaccine against it than one against smallpox.

Hepatitis

Superficially, infectious hepatitis (hepatitis B) has many similarities to AIDS. It is caused by a virus, and forms of hepatitis can result from contamination with parts of the virus. However, the hepatitis virus is probably more infectious than HIV; it seems to survive longer at low temperatures, and it may be infectious in smaller amounts.

During the 1960s and 1970s hepatitis was common among the staff of transplantation units. Like AIDS, hepatitis is transmitted in body fluids transferred between people; the most common vehicle is blood, and the most common pathway from a patient to a member of the medical or paramedical staff is by accidental contamination. At one time it appeared that hospital staff were more at risk than their patients.

AIDS, however, appears to carry little risk to hospital staff, though there have been a few isolated cases of infection. The epidemic of hepatitis resulted in an increased awareness of the risk to staff, and a revision of legislation and local regulation about the disposal of infected waste.

Hepatitis is now regarded as a serious venereal disease; its incubation period is short: 14 to 35 days.

Plague

Several public commentators have compared AIDS to the Black Death – a plague epidemic that ravaged Europe in the mid-fourteenth century and carried off a third of the population.

Plague, however, is caused by a bacillus, *Pasteurella pestis*, not by a virus. The bacillus lives in a primary host, usually the rat, in which it sometimes causes disease. This has been compared to the STLV-III virus in African green monkeys (see Chapter 4), but STLV-III is not HIV, and almost certainly does not cause disease in man.

The plague bacillus was transferred from rats to people by fleas, which feed indiscriminately on the blood of either. There is some comparison with AIDS in that HIV can live for an hour or more in bedbugs, which may transfer it from person to person. However, this is not a significant route of infection. The pneumonic form of plague was transmitted in droplets from the lungs and throat.

The incubation time of plague, and the interval from sickness to death, was a matter of days, whereas the incubation period of AIDS is a matter of years and the interval from sickness to death is a matter of months or a few years.

2 'It can't happen to me'

AIDS can afflict anyone who is infected with HIV by another person. HIV is carried in body fluids, so if you receive body fluid from an infected person – especially through sex, or by sharing needles for injecting drugs – you are at risk of getting AIDS (see diagram on page 77). This chapter explains what 'risk' is, and discusses the high-risk groups of people: it also explains how to reduce the risk to yourself of 'catching' AIDS. We explain the spread of HIV from person to person at greater length in Chapter 7, after we have described the virus and the disease in more detail.

What is risk?
The word 'risk' is bandied about in AIDS discussions – so much so that we need to define it. So far as this book is concerned, the word 'risk' has two meanings: first, it is a technical term used by statisticians; second, it refers to how the facts behind the statistics affect the individual. The sense in which we use the word should be clear in context.

Statisticians refer to 'groups' of people: all those people with something in common. For example, the group 'drug addicts' consists of all those people who are addicted to drugs. In order to study a group, a statistician selects a small number of people (a sample) from the group. The larger the sample, the more representative it is of the group. The smaller the sample, the less representative it is of the group.

To calculate the risk of AIDS in a group of people, such as drug addicts, the statistician will select a sample of people from the group, and a similar sample from another group, such as Britons, which includes the first group. Each subject in the first sample is classified as positive or negative for some factor (such as receptive anal intercourse) and as positive or negative for a disease state (such as developing AIDS). The formula for Relative risk is then applied; this gives a value for the risk, so that different groups of people can be compared.

High-risk groups

People in some groups are more likely to get AIDS than are people in other groups. The following is a widely accepted list of groups of people who, until recently, have been at high risk of getting AIDS:

- homosexual and bisexual men
- intravenous drug abusers
- haemophiliacs
- sexual partners of the above people
- infants born to infected mothers.

Within each group, the chance of an individual getting AIDS is variable. Consider, for example, the group 'homosexual men'. Were a particular homosexual man to have upward of a dozen, possibly even 30 homosexual partners each day (as was the practice for some homosexuals in New York, San Francisco and Los Angeles), then it would be very likely that he would catch HIV from at least one of his partners. But if another homosexual man had been faithful to one partner, and vice versa, for many years, then neither could catch HIV from the other (unless one caught the virus in a completely different way – from a blood transfusion, for example). So it is quite possible that someone in a high-risk group is actually not at risk of 'catching' AIDS.

Because of the variability between individuals within groups, we prefer another list of groups of people who are at high risk of becoming infected with HIV:

- People whose sexual partners were carrying HIV at the time of intercourse.
- People who have received blood, or blood products (or other body tissue or fluid), from a donor with HIV.
  You could come into the second category if you are:
  – haemophiliac

- someone who shares intravenous injection needles with other people
- a recipient of blood transfusions, organ transplants, skin grafts or artificial insemination.

● Babies born of mothers with HIV. We discuss this in more detail in Chapter 7.

There are very many groups in which people can be placed, and each person can be placed in several groups. A woman might be a lesbian and a drug addict. The risk of a lesbian catching HIV is very small; however, the risk of a drug addict catching HIV is high, and if she belongs to the group of addicts who share needles and syringes, then the risk is very high indeed. See diagram below. In the next part of this chapter we examine some of these high-risk groups, and explain why the people in them are at risk. There is one central theme: the transfer of body fluid from one person to another. The amount of body fluid appears not to be important; what *is* important is the number of infectious particles in the fluid. A smear of blood on a used razor blade or needle may be enough. A smear of vaginal fluid may be enough. In one case an unknown amount of an unknown body fluid from an AIDS patient entered the open sores of eczema on a nurse's hands, and thus transferred the infection.

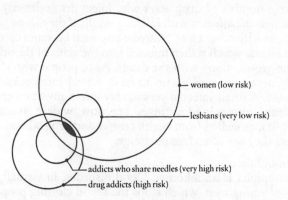

Not everyone who belongs to a risk group is at the same risk of AIDS as all the other people in that group. Although lesbians are at very low risk, a lesbian drug addict who shares needles (black overlap) is at very high risk. This diagram shows the relationships between these groups. (The areas of the circles are not to scale.)

Homosexual and bisexual men

The vast majority of AIDS sufferers are homosexual men. This is not because of their sexual orientation in itself, but because of the widespread promiscuity among certain groups of homosexual men before the nature and implications of AIDS became known. Once introduced to a gay community, the virus spread very quickly, especially in the big cities in America. By using the word 'promiscuous' we don't mean to be derogatory or judgemental, but simply indicate relative numbers of sexual partners. Thus, the more promiscuous a man is, the more likely he is to meet a sexual partner who is infected with HIV, and a more promiscuous man can pass the infection on to more partners than a less promiscuous man. See the diagram on page 77.

A man can transfer HIV in seminal fluid, and possibly in urine and faeces. Thus, a man who receives seminal fluid into his mouth or rectum from other, infected, men is very likely to become infected with HIV, not to mention gonorrhoea, syphilis and other venereal diseases. However, it has been proved that a man who ejaculates semen into other men, and does not receive any, is much less likely to become infected with HIV, and slightly less likely to catch some other venereal infections.

Intravenous drug abusers

A large number of drug users who inject drugs directly into their veins become infected with HIV, especially if they share needles and syringes with other users. Shared equipment becomes contaminated with blood, which is then injected into the veins of the other people in the group, along with the drugs. Also, people who share drugs equipment may well go on to have sexual intercourse with one another. A single infected person may infect any number of others.

Clean needles and syringes are now widely available from chemists, as well as from health centres and drug addiction centres, where they are often free of charge.

Haemophiliacs

Haemophilia is an inherited blood disorder, in virtually all cases only affecting men, which stops the blood clotting properly when exposed to the air. In severe cases, a haemophiliac can bleed to death. At present, the only treatment is periodic infusion of clotting Factors derived from donated blood.

By the start of 1988 some 20,000 haemophiliacs worldwide were infected with HIV, having been administered, unknowingly, with infected blood or blood products; 1,012 of these are in Britain. Since July 1985, however, only heat-treated blood products have been used in the treatment of haemophilia, and the risk of these blood products containing HIV is very low. Figures for the percentage of haemophiliacs who were infected with HIV between 1981 and 1985 vary, depending on the country, from 40 per cent to 90 per cent.

Children born of infected mothers
Transmission of HIV from infected mothers to their foetuses has now been proven. Up to 65 per cent of infected women infect their foetuses in the womb, but up to 95 per cent of infants born to infected mothers become infected. Most doctors now assume that babies born of infected mothers are already infected, until proved otherwise.

Doctors in many countries have advised infected women to consider being sterilised, to avoid the possibility of pregnancy. They advise infected pregnant women to have abortions, because of the near certainty of their bearing infected infants. So far, virtually all infected babies have developed AIDS within two years.

Risk of infection to people not in high-risk groups
The medical professions
So far very few people in the medical professions have become infected with HIV through their professional contact with AIDS patients. Transfer of infection via body fluids has been known about for over a century, and training is geared to prevent infection spreading. However, transmission of HIV to those caring for AIDS patients cannot be ruled out, as the case history overleaf shows.

The emergency services
Ambulance crews and police officers are exposed to body fluids in situations which are less controlled than in a hospital or an operating theatre. At the scene of an accident or a crime, body fluids such as blood, vomit, urine, faeces and seminal fluid may be present, perhaps in unexpected places. Emergency service crews are concerned primarily with saving life or containing crime. Protecting themselves – which includes protecting themselves from infectious body fluids – is a secondary consideration. However, in the year up to June 1987 emergency service crews were retrained, and they have been issued with special protective equipment.

Resuscitation of accident victims, though, is acknowledged to be dangerous in the light of AIDS; in particular, mouth-to-mouth resuscitation may bring the helper into contact with blood, vomit and other fluids. Ambulance crews now use special tubes to blow air into a victim's lungs: these keep the mouth and nose away from those of the victim.

CASE HISTORY

In the mid-1980s a white woman living in Africa had an attack of shingles. The next year she had severe inflammation of the mouth. The following year she came to a British hospital with general malaise, a dry cough and fever. She was given penicillin and recovered, but four weeks later had a high fever and difficulty in breathing. She had *P. carinii* pneumonia and, after intensive investigation for other causes, AIDS was diagnosed. She later died.

A nurse, taking a sample of blood during the investigations, accidentally stabbed herself with the needle, and infected herself with a droplet of the patient's blood. Thirteen days later she had a flu-like illness, with sore throat, headache, aching muscles, facial neuralgia and swollen glands. Four days later a rash spread over her chest, trunk, neck and face, and lasted for seven days. She was feverish up to 39°C until the twentieth day of the illness (33 days after the stab) after which she recovered.

Blood taken 27 days after the injury was negative for HIV, but was positive 49 days after. Her illness was caused by HIV.

Prostitutes

Prostitutes – women and men – receive seminal fluid from a range of men. Unless they use condoms, the more clients they have, the more likely they are to come into direct contact with venereal infections, including HIV.

Some prostitutes are also drug addicts – they may even have resorted to prostitution in order to finance their addiction. Many drug-addicted prostitutes are already infected with HIV: those who are not already infected are at great risk from infected clients and from infected shared needles and syringes. Drug-addicted prostitutes tend not to protect themselves against venereal diseases. Non-addicted female prostitutes and (in countries such as West Germany) licensed prostitutes usually protect themselves against venereal diseases with condoms: very few of these women are infected with HIV.

The armed forces
When soldiers go on leave they enjoy themselves, often with local prostitutes: this exposes them to venereal infections, including HIV.

Schoolteachers
Schoolteachers are exposed to all the contagious infections carried by their pupils – measles, mumps, glandular fever and so on. HIV, however, is not contagious, so teachers are no more likely to contract HIV than anyone else, and even then, only in the ways we have already described.

How to prevent it happening to you
Safe sex
Sexual intercourse is one hundred per cent safe only with someone who is not infected. The more sexual partners you have, the greater the risk of becoming infected. But if you have only one partner, and he or she has more than one, your risk increases. A prospective sexual partner may not know whether he or she has HIV – and may not want to find out.

You can be sure that you are not infected if you have two tests for HIV antibody, three months apart, and if you do not have sex between the two tests. The reasons for needing two tests, and for the time interval, are made clear in Chapter 9.

The idea that there is such a thing as 'safe sex' has become something of a cult. Partners stimulate one another by touching and stroking, but without sexual intercourse or internal ejaculation. Partners masturbate themselves, or one another, taking care that neither seminal fluid nor vaginal fluid comes into contact with the other person. However, practices such as insertion of an uncovered penis, fisting (inserting an uncovered fist into the anus), rimming (stimulating the anus with the lips or tongue), deep kissing, and mutual masturbation, should not be regarded as completely safe in terms of HIV transmission, if either partner is infected.

Condoms are becoming more widely used to reduce the risk of transferring body fluid. Using a condom is significantly safer than unprotected intercourse, but condoms occasionally tear and are often used incorrectly.

Condoms intended for family planning are not designed for anal intercourse: their failure rate during anal intercourse is significantly higher than during vaginal intercourse. Special condoms designed for anal intercourse are now available.

Notwithstanding all this, the safest course is to refrain from

23

sexual intercourse with an infected person.

Do not confuse contraception with preventing the transmission of virus. For example, a vasectomy is an effective form of contraception, but it will not prevent the transfer of infected seminal fluid; neither will the coil or the pill, though they are effective forms of contraception.

Safe blood

If you need a blood transfusion, the transfusion service will have checked that the blood contains no antibodies against HIV; by inference, they assume it does not contain the virus. However, if by chance infected blood was given while the donor was incubating HIV, virus will be present, but tests for antibody may be negative. In all, though, the risk of receiving infected blood is now extremely small: the National Blood Transfusion Service estimates the risk as less than one in five million.

The safest possible blood is your own. If you plan to go into hospital, perhaps for surgery, some Regional Transfusion Centres and some private companies will store some of your own blood in case it should be needed.

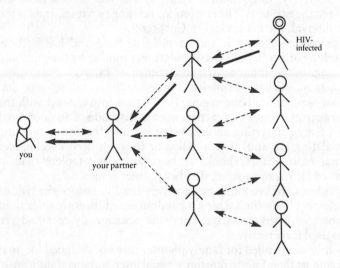

HIV-infected

you

your partner

However faithful you are, your partner's sexual contacts could kill you. The double-headed arrows show sexual relationships – the dark arrows show possible routes of infection.

A few Centres, and several private companies, offer to store your blood indefinitely. However, blood stored for longer than 28 days must be separated into plasma and cells, and the two components frozen. Thawing the frozen blood may take two hours or more and so it may not be available in emergencies. Moreover, the frozen blood would have to be transported to your emergency – which could take several hours and be very costly.

Safe blood products
If you have haemophilia your Association will have given you advice and information; if not, ask for it. Reducing, or delaying, your infusion therapy will not reduce your infection risks significantly, and may increase the risk of a dangerous bleed. Pasteurised infusions are safer than untreated infusion fluids, but do not try to pasteurise infusions yourself.

For people with haemophilia, the danger of infection with HIV has diminished considerably. The Transfusion Centres are aware of the risk and test all donors. The tests are becoming more reliable and more accurate, as are other methods of screening out infected donors. Purification and treatment of infusion fluids is improving, and Factors are safer now than they have ever been. It is also possible that haemophiliacs have a lower chance of developing AIDS than almost anyone else; see Chapter 7. Blood and blood products are discussed in more detail in Chapters 4 and 6.

Safe nursing
Professional nurses are trained to prevent the transfer of infection, and taught how to take blood and to clean patients safely. If you have no nursing training, but want to care for someone infected with HIV, or with AIDS, ask for professional help and advice. The

---

CASE HISTORY

A 36-year-old haemophiliac man, with HIV in his blood, had a motor accident and sustained brain damage. He became violent, and bit and scratched the people who cared for him. His mouth was frequently full of saliva and blood, and his fingernails constantly soiled with semen, faeces and urine.

Over a two-year period he bit and scratched 30 people, causing skin wounds which left residual scars; none of them became ill, and all were HIV-free six months after injury.

---

first person to approach is your family doctor: he or she may refer you directly to a source of help, such as a district nurse, or to one of the special help groups. Many of these are listed in Chapter 12 and any of them will advise you.

Safe first aid
The ability to give first aid to an accident victim is a matter of training and practice. Unfortunately, an untrained person can sometimes do more harm than good.

The priorities are:

● restore the heartbeat
● restore breathing
● stop any loss of blood.

Any danger of HIV transmission is in the last two of these. The most efficient way to restore breathing is mouth-to-mouth resuscitation – provided that it is carried out correctly – but the mouth and face of an accident victim may be covered in blood and vomit. If the victim is infected with HIV or has AIDS, the virus can be transferred to you by the blood. Remember that while the likelihood of an accident victim having AIDS is very low, the chance that he or she is infected with HIV is tenfold higher.

The correct form of mouth-to-mouth resuscitation does not result in inhaling or swallowing the victim's blood or saliva. If the victim's injuries allow it, another method of artificial respiration could be used.

Stopping the loss of blood from an injury is straightforward, but the first aider almost always becomes stained. Keep the blood away from cuts or wounds elsewhere on your body.

The Red Cross and the St John Ambulance Brigade will teach you to give first aid safely.

Safe social contact
You are in no danger of catching HIV from infected people or from AIDS patients during normal social contact. Handshakes, cheek kissing, and so on will not transfer the virus. The same applies to working together, provided that you do not come into contact with their body fluids.

Safe injection
If you inject drugs regularly or often, your immune response may be lower than normal, and you may become infected more easily. You

should avoid close associations, especially sexual intercourse, with infected people. If you inject drugs, always use new, clean equipment for mixing, cutting and injecting. Never borrow equipment from someone else. Never inject drugs that someone else has mixed or cut with their equipment.

The use of drugs not prescribed by a doctor is not safe. The behaviour which follows the use of drugs can result in accidents causing injury or death; the drugs themselves can cause serious illness and death.

Try this questionnaire. There is no scoring system, but the more times you answer YES, the more likely you are to be at risk from AIDS.

Have you had more than five sexual partners in the last five years?	YES/NO
Do you use hard drugs?	YES/NO
Do you inject drugs?	YES/NO
Do you share your injection equipment with other people?	YES/NO
Has your partner had more than five other partners in the last five years?	YES/NO
Do you suffer from haemophilia?	YES/NO
Do you use blood products more than five times weekly?	YES/NO
Have you had any of the following in the last five years?	
Blood transfusions	
Kidney transplant	
Skin graft	
Artificial insemination	YES/NO
Are you a homosexual man?	YES/NO
Do you receive seminal fluid into your rectum or mouth?	YES/NO
Have you had more than five sexual partners in the last five weeks?	YES/NO
Do you ever have sex with more than one person in one day?	YES/NO

---

3 AIDS – Some questions & answers

When people knew very little about AIDS all sorts of tales arose, and were passed around as if they were true. In this chapter we examine, in the light of our present understanding, some of the questions which have troubled people.

'Does kissing spread AIDS?'
HIV has occasionally been recovered from the saliva of infected people. The tonsils may be a reservoir of and a nursery for the virus. However, the saliva of some people may contain one or more substances which inactivate HIV. There are no documented cases of the transmission of HIV by saliva, but it is possible that, if enough saliva containing enough virus were transferred from one person to another, HIV could be transmitted in this way.

Social kissing does not spread HIV: lightly touching another person's cheek, hand or lips with your lips will not spread HIV. It is not known whether more intimate kissing can do so. Prolonged French kissing – where one person's tongue is inserted into another person's mouth – may transfer saliva from one person to another. Kissing other parts of the body, such as the penis, vulva or anus, may result in an exchange of body fluids. If one person is infected with HIV, the other may catch it.

The issue is confused because intimate kissing is often followed by sexual intercourse or by mutual masturbation, and HIV is known to be transmitted in seminal fluid.

Kissing open sores or wounds, such as when a mother 'kisses it better' is perfectly safe when neither person is infected with HIV, but may spread the virus if either person is infected.

'Can lavatory seats, hand towels, cutlery and crockery spread AIDS?'
HIV is a fragile virus, and is destroyed by heating, cooling or drying. A cleaned, dry lavatory seat is therefore safe.

A lavatory seat – or, indeed, any other surface – bearing recently spilled body fluid containing HIV could transmit the virus if the fluid were to enter the body of another person.

The same is true for hand towels, cutlery and crockery, as well as shared drinking vessels, whether a chalice or a celebratory champagne bottle.

'Can sharing wind instruments spread AIDS?'
Unlikely unless enough body fluid were transferred.

'Can swimming pools and public baths spread AIDS?'
The water in public swimming pools is treated with chlorine or iodine to kill bacteria and viruses but, at the concentrations used, HIV might not be completely destroyed for several hours.

If virus were released from an infected person into a swimming pool it would be diluted: it is very unlikely that anyone would 'catch AIDS' in this way.

The water in public baths and showers is not reused before treatment which would kill infective virus. In communal baths the use of soaps and detergents would kill any virus in the water. However, showers are safer in this respect than communal baths.

Jacuzzis are more likely to be infected with other organisms, such as some bacteria, than with HIV, but they are a potential, though unlikely, source of cross-infection.

Between 1979 and 1986 the San Francisco bathhouses were a major source of infection, but this is because they were meeting places for homosexual men who transferred the virus during homosexual intercourse.

'Does having antibody in your blood mean you will develop AIDS?'
Most people who have antibody against HIV eventually get AIDS. The average incubation period (from becoming infected with HIV to having AIDS) is about five years, but it can be less than one year. AIDS has been recognised only since 1979. Time alone will tell how

long the incubation period might be, and what percentage of infected people go on to develop AIDS.

There are no recorded cases of anyone who has the virus later becoming virus-free. If you are seropositive – that is, if your blood contains antibody against HIV – you may develop AIDS during or after your next viral, bacterial, fungal or parasitic infection.

'Can babies get AIDS from their mothers?'

It is very likely that women who carry the virus will transmit it to their babies, and it is almost certain that those babies will go on to develop AIDS. Women who carry the virus can transmit it to their babies through the placenta during pregnancy, through vaginal secretions and blood during delivery, or from milk during breast-feeding. Newborn infants become infected and develop AIDS much more easily than do other people. Up to 65 per cent of infected women transmit HIV to their foetuses in the womb, and up to 95 per cent of babies born to infected mothers eventually become infected. Virtually all infected babies develop AIDS or ARC (AIDS-Related Complex) within two years.

'Do haemophiliacs spread AIDS?'

Haemophiliacs who are infected with HIV or who have AIDS do not spread it in some mysterious way unknown to other people. Haemophilia is characterised by the loss or impairment of the normal clotting ability of blood; haemophiliacs therefore rely on infusions of Factors derived from blood to survive.

Up to 1986, many haemophiliacs became infected with HIV from infected blood products. They were (and still are) capable of transmitting the virus to their sexual partners. Those who have not become infected won't spread it.

'Do only gays get AIDS?'

Men and women can become infected whether they are heterosexual, bisexual or homosexual. The virus passes from a sexual partner who carries it, by vaginal, anal or (possibly) oral sex.

Infants may become infected from their virus-carrying mothers, through the placenta during pregnancy, or from vaginal secretions and blood at delivery, or from milk during breast-feeding.

Intravenous drug-users who share injection equipment can become infected – the virus is transmitted in smears and drops of blood when equipment is shared.

Anyone who becomes infected is likely to go on to get AIDS.

e blood donors at risk?'

ou cannot become infected with HIV by giving blood. The transfusion services of most developed countries do not re-use needles, blood lines or other equipment.

In all developed countries blood donors are tested for HIV antibodies when they give blood. If the test is positive, they may be told this, and may be informed of the risks of developing AIDS and of transmitting HIV.

In some developing countries needles may be re-used, and may not be properly cleaned between donors. The virus may be transmitted from one donor to another via dirty needles.

'Can women get AIDS from men?'

Men who are infected with HIV carry the virus in cells in their seminal fluid: it can be transferred to women during vaginal and anal sex, and possibly during oral sex, and can result in AIDS.

'Can men get AIDS from women?'

Women with HIV have been shown to carry the virus in the cells in vaginal and cervical secretions, albeit in only small amounts, but the vagina and cervix therefore provide a source of virus for transmission to male sexual partners. There are many documented cases of men getting HIV infection, which may develop into AIDS, from women.

In many parts of Central Africa equal numbers of men and women (up to 35 per cent in some age groups) are infected with HIV. It is possible (but unlikely) that up to 35 per cent of the men are receptive homosexuals; it is more likely that the virus is passed equally easily between the sexes in either direction.

'Do condoms prevent the transmission of the virus?'

The virus will not pass through an intact condom; however, condoms do fail. Fifteen per cent of women whose partners use condoms as the only means of contraception become pregnant within one year. Condoms tear, slip, or are used incorrectly. It follows that women whose infected partners use condoms to avoid transmitting HIV may be at some risk.

It is likely that up to 50 per cent of contraceptive condoms fail (by damage or misuse) during anal intercourse. Special condoms are available for anal intercourse: they reduce the risk of infection markedly, but not completely.

The use of condoms must therefore not be thought of, or described as, truly 'safe sex'.

'Is AIDS spread by coughing and sneezing?'
There is no evidence for the spread of HIV by coughs and sneezes. However, if enough spray containing enough virus is transferred from one person to another, the infection could be transferred too.

'Can you catch AIDS at the dentist?'
Dentists are at some risk of catching HIV from infected patients if enough blood – or possibly enough saliva – containing enough virus is transferred.

Dirty dental instruments can carry HIV in the same way that dirty injection needles can, but reputable dentists do not re-use anaesthetic needles or syringes. They clean their instruments by scrubbing or wiping them with water and a detergent. Most dentists also sterilise them by soaking in a fluid such as sodium hypochlorite solution, or by autoclaving at a high temperature and pressure.

If you have any doubts, ask your dentist how the instruments are cleaned and sterilised, and whether needles or syringes are re-used.

'Can you catch AIDS at the acupuncturist, ear-piercer, hairdresser or tattooist?'
Again, if enough infected body fluid were transferred to the client, there might be a risk, but we know of no recorded case of AIDS resulting from any of these practices.

'Can you catch AIDS by being near someone with AIDS or someone infected with HIV?'
No, you can't. You need to transfer body fluid before you are at any risk.

'Can you catch AIDS by sharing a toothbrush or razor?'
Gums bleed; razors nick. If you use an infected person's toothbrush or razor after that person, there is a chance of your becoming infected. If you clean the toothbrush or razor thoroughly, you reduce the chance of becoming infected.

'Was the AIDS virus man-made in a laboratory . . . ?'
There's no evidence for this.

' . . . or did it come from outer space?'
The evidence for the origin of viruses from outer space is slim, and not widely believed.

'Can mouth-to-mouth resuscitation spread AIDS?'
If enough body fluid were transferred from an infected person the

virus could be spread. The correct form of mouth-to-mouth resuscitation does not result in inhaling or swallowing the victim's blood or saliva. Look again at Chapter 2, where we discuss 'safe first aid'. Ambulances carry special equipment to safeguard the crew from the victim – and the victim from the crew.

'Can mingling blood as a blood brother or sister spread AIDS?'
This is clearly a dangerous practice – if present, HIV will almost certainly be transferred from one to another.

'Can people who work with AIDS sufferers catch AIDS?'
People who care for AIDS patients very rarely catch the virus, but there are a few recorded cases. These have resulted from a breakdown in the usual precautions for handling infected patients and waste material – most of them because of an accidental stabbing with a needle used for taking blood from an infected person.

People who work alongside HIV-infected people are not at risk if they practise normal standards of cleanliness and hygiene. There is a risk if an infected person has an accident or becomes ill and if body fluid is spilled.

'Can artificial insemination cause AIDS?'
If a woman were artificially inseminated with sperm from an HIV-infected donor, she would be very likely to become infected, and to develop AIDS. However, as all sperm donated to sperm banks since 1986 has been tested for HIV, the likelihood of a woman becoming infected in this way is less than it was.

'Can organ transplants cause AIDS?'
A number of transplant recipients have become infected with HIV from donated tissue – such as kidneys and skin – from infected donors. If the donor were infected then, in theory, any transplant (heart, lung, kidney, cornea, skin) or donation of blood or semen could transmit HIV to the recipient who might then develop AIDS. In developed countries all donors are now tested for HIV.

'Are tests for AIDS reliable?'
The usual screening tests for the presence of antibody against HIV are about 90 per cent reliable. A few results will be falsely positive (see Chapter 9).

A few people (especially babies) develop AIDS without having had any detectable antibody. Any positive test for antibody should be followed by several other tests to confirm the result. Reasons for any discrepancies should be discovered.

Tests for active virus are not widely available, and are often falsely negative (see Chapter 9).

'Can other people catch the opportunistic infections that an AIDS patient has?'
The opportunistic infections of AIDS include *Pneumocystis carinii*, mycobacterium, cytomegalovirus (CMV), cryptosporidium, candida (thrush) and many other bacteria, viruses, fungi and parasites (see Chapter 5).

These organisms are all around us and often cause transient infectious illnesses. The severity of the illness depends on the state of a person's health. Many healthy people are infected over a long period with some of these organisms, but they do not become ill unless or until the immune system is depressed.

'Has the advice to football clubs been too severe?'
The Football Association, and many clubs, have suggested that players should not share baths; they should not drink from the same cups or bottles; they should not share clothing, combs, razors; the bucket and sponge should be replaced by antiseptics, cotton wool and waterproof plasters. The advice is based on good hygiene.

'Can tampons and sanitary towels spread AIDS?'
The blood on tampons and sanitary towels used by infected women contains HIV. If the virus in that blood gets into another person, that other person may become infected.

Used towels and liners should be placed in a bag and burned immediately; tampons may be flushed down the lavatory immediately after removal. Spills or drips should be cleaned with a household bleach or strong detergent.

People who have to empty sanitary bins should wear rubber gloves. They should burn the contents or treat it with strong household bleach. The bin should then be washed with a solution of bleach.

'Can lesbians catch AIDS?'
Lesbians can 'catch AIDS' if they receive body fluid from an HIV-infected person. However, women who have sexual relations only with other women are unlikely to 'catch AIDS' through their sexual activities. They are as likely as anyone else to do so from dirty injection needles, and so on. A lesbian whose sexual partner has AIDS or HIV is more likely to become infected and develop AIDS than one whose partner does not have AIDS.

'Can HIV be carried in food?'
Very unlikely.

'Has AIDS been around for a hundred years?'
Probably not. But forms of the virus very similar to HIV have been around for a long time – possibly as long as man. Viruses mutate. The current strain of HIV has evolved to overcome the resistance of its hosts – human beings.

4   The Human Immunodeficiency Virus

What is a virus?

A virus is an infectious particle, partly a living creature and partly a non-living chemical, too small to be seen with an optical microscope.

A virus is far smaller than a bacterium. Bacteria can be seen with the aid of an optical microscope and can be trapped in very fine filters. Viruses, by contrast, pass through all known filters, and can be seen only by using the much higher magnification of an electron microscope.

Bacteria live and reproduce on surfaces, or as particles in suspension, floating in a fluid such as blood or urine. Viruses, on the other hand, can live and reproduce only inside another living cell. Outside a cell, in the blood or in the urine, a virus is an inert collection of chemicals that cannot feed or reproduce, and which dissolves in the fluid, just as does salt or sugar.

The two main chemicals that make up a virus are protein and nucleic acid. The protein forms a coat, or envelope, around the core of the virus; the nucleic acid is contained in the core. There are two kinds of nucleic acid, ribonucleic acid and deoxyribonucleic acid, abbreviated to RNA and DNA. Singly or together, RNA and DNA form the genes of all animals, plants, bacteria and viruses. In all animal and plant cells, DNA forms the complex centre of the chromosomes, and carries all the information which a cell needs to carry out all its processes. The information is copied, or transcribed, in small pieces, on to strands of RNA which, in their turn, use the information to make proteins, and enzymes, which carry out the processes of life.

The nucleic acid of a virus is very similar to that of an animal or plant; it carries the genes for the virus, providing the information about the shape and structure of the protein envelope, the composition of the nucleic acid, the method by which the virus enters a cell and the instructions for making new viruses. Most of the viruses that infect animals have DNA in their core; most of those that infect plants have RNA in their core.

Outside a host cell, the nucleic acid of a virus is a non-living chemical; once inside such a cell, it tells the cell to make many copies of the invading virus. Following instructions, the cell produces both virus protein and virus nucleic acid: it then assembles them into viruses, possibly as many as a thousand copies per cell, and releases them into the fluid surrounding itself. During the release of new viruses, the cell may burst and die: if it does the virus is said to be cytopathic (from the Greek *cyto* – a cell, and *pathos* – suffering). If the cell does not die it may continue to make new viruses while its own life processes continue at a reduced rate. Some viruses remain dormant inside cells for years, even decades, before the cells begin to make copies.

Human Immunodeficiency Virus
The nucleic acid in the core of HIV is RNA, not DNA. When HIV enters a human cell the information in the RNA is transcribed into the DNA of the host cell by an enzyme called reverse transcriptase (RT). The new DNA then becomes incorporated into the chromosome of the cell. Viruses which do this are called retroviruses. The presence of RT activity has become an accepted sign of the presence of a retrovirus; very often the type of RT activity indicates which retrovirus is present.

The new DNA instructs the host cell to make many replica viruses, identical to the first. These eventually move to the surface of, and leave, the cell, wrapping themselves in an extra envelope of proteins from components of the host cell's membrane. As the new viruses leave the host cell, it dies. The new viruses, now free in the body fluid, are ready to infect many more cells.

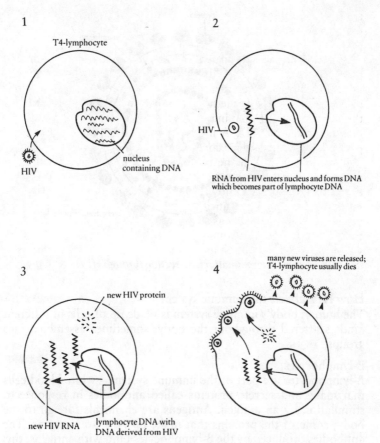

The cycle of replication of HIV. For explanation see overleaf.

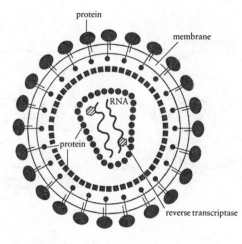

Diagrammatic cross-section through HIV.

How HIV affects the immune system
The human body's immune system is made up of cells of different kinds scattered throughout the body, sometimes assembled into groups.

B-lymphocytes
B-lymphocytes are part of the immune system – white blood cells that make and secrete proteins called antibodies in response to stimulation by an antigen. Antigens are chemicals foreign to the body; some of the proteins that make up HIV are antigens. The antibodies produced by the B-lymphocytes bind with antigens; this binding sometimes results in the inactivation of the virus or bacterium of which the antigen is part. It is not yet clear whether this is so for HIV.

B-lymphocytes move freely in the blood, but are more or less fixed in the lymph nodes, spleen and various other lymphoid organs (see diagram).

T-lymphocytes
T-lymphocytes are also cells that play a part in the immune system. There are at least two forms: T4-lymphocytes (also called helper cells) help B-lymphocytes to recognise antigens; without them, particular antibodies might not be produced. T4-lymphocytes are

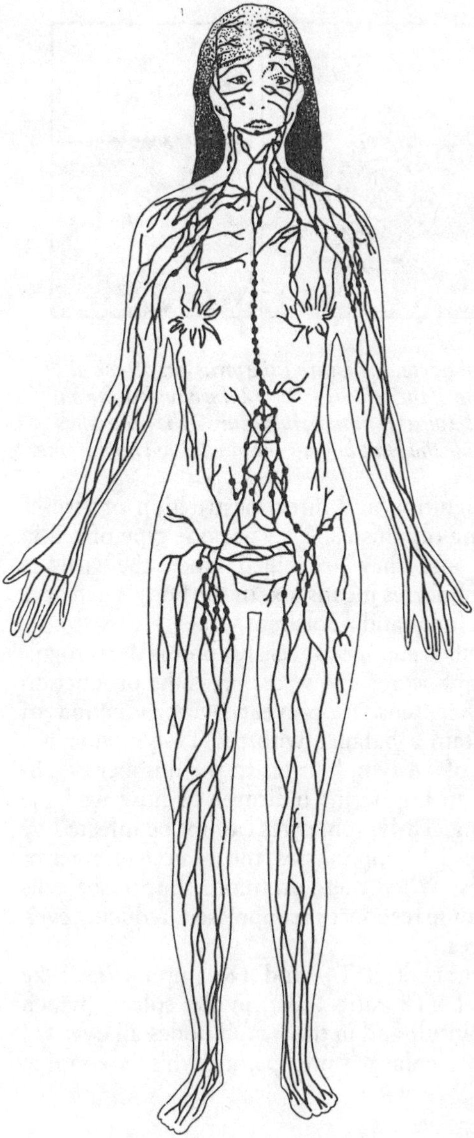

This shows the lymphatic system, a network of channels similar to blood vessels, that covers all the body's organs, except the nervous system. The vessels drain lymph, a yellowish watery fluid derived from blood, out of the infinitesimally small spaces between cells to a blood vessel in the neck. At intervals on the lymph network there are lymph glands – also called nodes and shown here as dots – which act as filters in certain parts of the body. It is here that immune defence cells called lymphocytes destroy bacteria in the lymph before it is drained back into the blood. Lymph nodes swell up and became tender when the lymphocytes are infected with certain types of virus, including HIV – this is lymphadenopathy (see page 55).

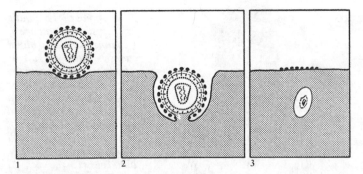

Entry of HIV into a T4-lymphocyte. In picture 1 the virus has attached itself to the surface membrane of the cell. In picture 2 the lymphocyte has formed a pouch into which the virus is drawn. In picture 3 the pouch has sealed off and the virus is inside the lymphocyte, within its own membrane.

also involved in the recognition and direct destruction of viruses and other antigen-carrying organisms. They are one type of cell in which HIV reproduces, and they are killed when the virus is released. Loss of T4-lymphocytes means loss of the body's defences against viruses, bacteria, fungi and parasites.

T8-lymphocytes (also called suppressor cells) suppress the recognition of antigens by B-lymphocytes and so suppress the production of specific antibody. They tend to prevent overproduction of antibody and they maintain a balance with the T4-lymphocytes. The ratio of the number of T4-lymphocytes to the number of T8-lymphocytes (T4/T8) is an important indicator of how well the immune system is working. T8-lymphocytes cannot be infected by HIV. But as the virus kills T4-lymphocytes, the relative number of T8-lymphocytes increases. When there are more suppressor cells than helper cells, the immune response is suppressed, reducing even further the body's defences.

The changes in the numbers of T4- and T8-lymphocytes take place in the blood (the T4/T8 ratio falls), in the spleen (which becomes enlarged and painful) and in the lymph nodes all over the body (which also become enlarged and painful: this is lymphadenopathy).

Activation of lymphocytes

When any of these lymphocytes recognises a foreign protein (antigen) they become activated by it, that is, they increase in size and

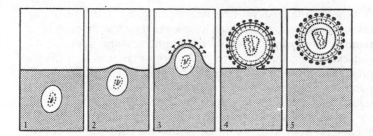

New viruses leaving a T4-lymphocyte. Pictures 1–4 show the formation of a protein envelope, derived from the outer membrane of the lymphocyte. Picture 5 shows a complete virus, after separating from the lymphocyte.

reproduce many times, so that there is a large increase in the numbers of antigen-recognising lymphocytes. Some of the new B-lymphocytes become non-replicating plasma cells, which then make antibody. Others go on replicating to increase the numbers. Others stop replicating and become memory cells – that is, they are dormant until they are again exposed to the specific antigen that activated them.

Lymphocytes become activated in response to any kind of antigen, from an infection, from a transplanted organ or from an allergy. It is likely that HIV will bind to and enter only activated T4-lymphocytes.

Activation by antigen affects only those B-lymphocytes and T-lymphocytes which are programmed to recognise that antigen. Some viruses, such as the Epstein–Barr virus, which causes glandular fever, activate all B-lymphocytes, whether they are programmed to recognise the antigens of the virus or not. Glandular fever, in which the lymph glands swell and become painful, is the result of widespread, non-specific activation and proliferation of B-lymphocytes.

People with chronically or frequently activated T-lymphocytes appear to become infected with HIV more easily than others. They may also develop AIDS more easily than others.

Like the Epstein–Barr virus, HIV causes activation of B-lymphocytes; however, HIV infection results not in glandular fever but in lymphadenopathy. The two illnesses have similar symptoms, but lymphadenopathy resulting from HIV infection is more persistent.

Another glandular-fever-like illness (caused by cytomegalovirus) is one of the infections to which homosexual men with AIDS often succumb. The lymphocytes of haemophiliacs and promiscuous homosexual men may be activated more often, and to a greater degree, than those of other people. Haemophiliacs are frequently exposed to large amounts of antigenic proteins through the blood products they need. Promiscuous homosexual men who take the receptive role in sex are exposed to large amounts of antigenic seminal fluid in the rectum. It may be that the lymphocytes of drug addicts are similarly activated by the milk powder with which they often 'cut' their drugs.

The people of central Africa are constantly exposed to a large number of viral, bacterial, fungal and parasitic infections. Many such people are infected at a subclinical level – that is, they show no symptoms – and their lymphocytes are permanently activated.

For example, in Zaire, people who have antibody against HIV often also have antibody against *Plasmodium falciparum*, which causes malaria. It is likely that infection with the malaria parasite causes an activation of T4-lymphocytes, which then become vulnerable to infection by HIV, should a person be exposed to the virus.

Macrophages
Macrophages, also part of the immune system, are cells that scavenge the entire body for debris, including antigenic particles. They work with T4-lymphocytes in presenting antigen to B-lymphocytes. Macrophages, too, can become infected with HIV, and may form reservoirs of virus in any part of the body, including the brain.

Isolating HIV

HIV can be propagated in certain human T-lymphocytes that have been adapted to grow under laboratory conditions.

In isolating virus from a patient, a sample of blood is separated to obtain the T-lymphocytes. These are then exposed to biochemicals that cause them to proliferate in culture in the laboratory. Virus released from the proliferating (and dying) T-lymphocytes is transferred into the laboratory-adapted T-lymphocytes, of which there are various kinds. One kind continues to proliferate in culture, even when infected with HIV; thus the virus is propagated at the same time as the T-lymphocytes. Another kind of modified T-lymphocyte is killed by the virus, and forms a characteristic, ring-shaped giant cell with many nuclei. This type of T-lymphocyte can be used to quantify the virus.

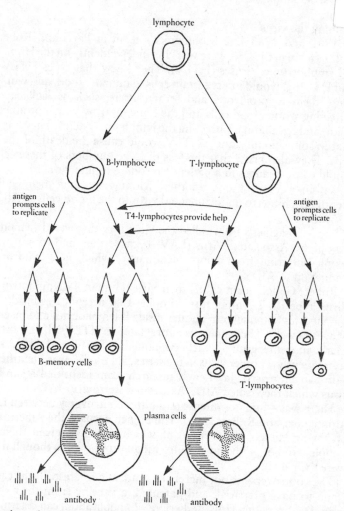

This shows how lymphocytes respond to antigens, such as those on viruses.
Lymphocytes from the bone marrow develop into B-lymphocytes and
T-lymphocytes. Both kinds are activated by antigen; they then replicate.
B-lymphocytes replicate to form many memory cells and some plasma cells.
The plasma cells make antibody which binds with the antigen which
activated the cells. The memory cells replicate to make plasma cells when
they next meet antigen. T-lymphocytes replicate to make many T-
lymphocytes which recognise that specific antigen.

Naming the virus

In 1982 and 1983 Luc Montagnier's team in Paris and Robert Gallo's team in the USA were working independently on the Human T-Lymphotropic Viruses (HTLV). They knew that types HTLV-I and HTLV-II would infect certain cells in human blood, and would cause them to proliferate and form cancers, such as leukaemias (affecting white blood cells and the bone marrow which produces them) and lymphomas (affecting the lymphatic system). They knew that in some circumstances HTLV would cause the death of these cells. They also knew that the loss of large numbers of these cells would cause changes in a patient's response to infections.

Within a year of one another, Montagnier and then Gallo identified a hitherto undocumented virus in the blood cells of AIDS patients.

Luc Montagnier's team called the virus they discovered Lymphadenopathy Associated Virus (LAV) because they had found it in people suffering from lymphadenopathy, which is a syndrome leading up to AIDS.

Robert Gallo's team called their virus Human T-Lymphotropic Virus, type III. T-lymphotropic implies that it replicates inside T-lymphocytes (although it replicates inside B-lymphocytes and macrophages as well). The name was abbreviated to HTLV-III, as it fitted neatly into the group which contained HTLV-I and HTLV-II. Subsequently, another virus in the series, HTLV-IV, was identified.

In San Francisco, Jay Levy's research team identified a similar virus which they called AIDS-Associated Retrovirus (ARV).

There was – and is – intense and bitter controversy between Luc Montagnier and Robert Gallo. The French accused the Americans of having 'stolen' their virus (of which they had given them a sample), and of publishing results and photographs as though they were their own.

The controversy is not merely of academic interest. Both teams claim to have prepared, and patented, a vaccine from their own virus. Discovery of a virus, and priority of publication, can determine ownership of patents for vaccines – and vaccines in this case could be worth a lot of money. Unfortunately, this wrangling delayed testing HIV vaccines.

The controversy was partially settled in March 1987, when the teams agreed to pool their patents and donate 80 per cent of their royalties to a newly formed research institute.

Because of the controversy, other scientists tended to refer to the new virus as HTLV-III/LAV. In 1986 an international committee suggested that it be called Human Immunodeficiency Virus (HIV) – the name we use in this book.

HIV, however, is not an entirely satisfactory name. It does not, for example, describe the nature of the virus, or its place among the viruses generally. Moreover, there are other forms of human immunodeficiency: congenital immunodeficiencies are not caused by a virus at all. Also, the related viruses HTLV-I and HTLV-II might, in some circumstances, cause immunological changes and deficiencies.

Infection with HIV

It is not yet clear how infectious HIV is. Almost certainly, different strains of virus affect people more or less easily, and the number of infectious particles transferred from person to person is significant. This depends partly on the number of infectious particles in the body fluid, and even more on whether the person being infected has bleeding cuts or weeping sores into which the virus can pass.

Different people seem to respond differently, and it is possible that some people, by virtue of their genetic make-up, are more easily infected than others. In addition, a person in poor health, or someone whose immune system is depressed, may be more easily infected than a healthy person.

Infection with HIV is often – though not always – followed by a flu-like illness, with headaches, fevers, chills, night sweats, muscle pains, rashes and transient swelling of lymph nodes.

This primary illness is not AIDS: it is an illness caused directly by HIV. It may be mild and transient; it may pass unnoticed. On the other hand it may last six weeks or longer and cause severe illness. In such cases it may be accompanied by lack of control of the muscles in the face or limbs, by red swollen rashes over the body, by brain damage and loss of emotional control (dementia), and by a reduction in the number of platelets and white cells in the blood, which results in bleeding from the skin and from mucous membranes, for instance the respiratory tract and the alimentary canal. When the primary illness is severe, and lasts a long time, it may overlap with AIDS, and it may be difficult to say which symptoms relate to which disease.

Most people, except perhaps infants, recover more or less completely from this primary illness. Those whose illness was severe may be left with some dementia. Many will have lymphadenopathy – swollen, painful and damaged lymph glands in many parts of the body, notably in the groin and armpits.

In most viral illnesses the meaning of the words 'incubation period' is clear; it is the time between infection and the appearance of signs and symptoms. In infections such as influenza, scarlet fever or smallpox, the incubation period is clearly defined to within a day or two, even to within a few hours.

For AIDS, the term 'incubation period' has been used in several ways, for instance to describe the interval between infection with HIV and the diagnosis of AIDS. In this sense, the incubation period of AIDS varies in different people from a few months to several years – possibly many years.

More specifically, the incubation period of HIV infection – that is, from infection to the appearance of symptoms of the primary illness – ranges from six days to three months, though it may be longer. At the longer time intervals it may not be clear whether the symptoms are associated with infection or with seroconversion, which we describe later.

After the primary illness, HIV can often be isolated from the T4-lymphocytes in the blood. Proteins and antigens characteristic of the virus may also be present in the blood. The number of T4-lymphocytes may be lower than normal, and the T4/T8 ratio may be low; this is typical of immunodeficiency. After the primary illness, many people are mildly immunodeficient; usually they do not have AIDS Related Complex (ARC – see page 55) or AIDS, though they may have lymphadenopathy.

A person is infectious any time after infection, and can transmit the virus to other people.

Seroconversion

Some time after the primary illness, most people produce antibody against HIV. This change (from having no antibody to having antibody) is known as seroconversion, and the patient becomes seropositive for HIV. This is the point at which a test for antibody against HIV would be positive. A small number of patients, including most babies, do not seroconvert (that is, do not produce antibodies).

Seroconversion may be accompanied by another flu-like illness, similar to the primary illness; it may be more or less severe in its effects, and has also been likened to glandular fever. In some people, seroconversion has damaged the brain, and they have experienced several weeks of fever, general malaise and changes of mood, sometimes accompanied by epileptic seizures.

After seroconversion the great majority of people remain sero-positive. Virus antigen is not usually detectable in their blood, but virus can often be isolated from their T-lymphocytes. There have been a very few cases of people who have again become seronegative and remained symptom-free.

In the late stages of HIV infection, virus can be isolated from virtually all organs of the body. During these late stages the amount of antibody in the blood falls and may become undetectable. Two suggestions have been made to explain this:

● immunodeficiency may have progressed to the point where antibody can no longer be produced
● the amount of virus in the body may be so great that all remaining antibody is mopped up.

Antibody may protect the patient, to some extent, against the spread of the virus and the onset of AIDS; once the antibody has disappeared, death from AIDS is imminent.

Strains of HIV
A virus is recognised partly by its appearance in the electron microscope, partly by the chemicals it contains (such as RNA, DNA or RT), partly by the antigens that it has (these are recognised in the laboratory by antibodies taken from people infected with the virus), and partly by the cells it infects and the illness it causes.

One of the problems in this field is that antigens are not unique to a particular virus, or strain of virus. Each virus has many (perhaps dozens) of antigens; a sample of the same virus taken from another person may have most of the antigens of the first sample, but may lack a few and have a few of its own. A different virus may have a few antigens in common with the first, but may lack/have many antigens that the first virus has/lacks.

This is why, if a person is infected with one virus, the antibodies that he or she makes against it may recognise other similar viruses, or even quite different viruses.

In the early years of the AIDS epidemic, researchers examined each patient, looking for viruses that might cause AIDS. By 1985 samples (called isolates) had been taken from about a hundred people with AIDS. The virus isolated from people in Paris was called LAV; those isolated from people in America were called HTLV-III and ARV. Comparisons of these isolates showed that they were sufficiently similar to be considered the same virus, but that there were differences. Most of the isolates were very similar; a few were a little different, perhaps different enough to be separate strains.

By 1986, three hundred isolates had been examined in detail, and sub-groups or strains of HIV had been identified; there were hints that some strains were local to particular geographical areas. It was also suggested that some strains might infect people more easily than others and that some might result in more severe diseases than others, but this has not been proved. If the latter turns out to be true, there is a possibility that a non-virulent strain could be isolated from people or animals for laboratory culture and used as a vaccine.

Strains and sub-groups of HIV differ from one another in small but measurable ways. The more different one strain is from another, the easier it is for tests to distinguish between them. When they are quite different they are different viruses, but the meaning of 'quite different' is the subject of discussion and controversy, even quarrelling, among scientists.

Similar viruses

Several other viruses have been discovered and described during the intense research on AIDS and HIV. Some of these may cause AIDS, others may not; any of these may provide clues to the origin of HIV. The study of them will almost certainly help in the search for a vaccine.

In 1985 a virus called HTLV-IV was discovered in African people with AIDS. It is not clear whether HTLV-IV causes AIDS, whether it occurs coincidentally in people with AIDS, or whether it is a modified form of HIV. HTLV-IV is more like the monkey virus Simian TLV-III than HIV, but the antibodies which patients make against it are picked up by the HIV screening tests. The antibodies can be differentiated only by more complex tests. In 1986, a virus very similar to HIV, and perhaps to HTLV-IV, was isolated from a serum sample collected from a healthy person in 1976.

During 1986, yet another virus, which was called LAV-II to distinguish it from the French LAV, was isolated from African patients with AIDS. LAV-II looks like HIV under the electron microscope. It attacks and kills T-lymphocytes in the same way, but has clear differences from HIV. It is unlikely that LAV-II has evolved from HIV in recent years: it may have been present in the Central African Republic since 1980 or earlier. Patients who have LAV-II seem to be infected with HIV as well, so it is not clear whether or not this virus causes AIDS.

In the continuing search for viruses that might cause AIDS, or that are similar to HIV, various groups of people in Venezuela were tested. HIV antigens, purified from the whole virus, were used in laboratory tests to recognise antibodies in the blood of Amazonian Indians, people with malaria, and healthy Venezuelans, Europeans and Americans.

A large proportion of the population was found to have antibodies which would bind, in laboratory tests, with antigens of HIV. But AIDS is rare in Venezuela and none of the people with antibody had AIDS or HIV. Searches eventually isolated an unusual retrovirus, which was named South American Retrovirus (SA-RV), from the people who had malaria. SA-RV shares many antigens with HIV; if the immune system makes antibodies against these antigens, the antibodies recognise both SA-RV and HIV. SA-RV has not yet been studied in detail, and it is not yet clear exactly how many antigens it shares with HIV, and how many are different. We don't yet know whether SA-RV causes AIDS (though it's unlikely), or indeed any disease. That it was found in patients with malaria is probably a coincidence.

A virus that is endemic in some colonies of healthy African green monkeys, Simian T-lymphotropic virus, type III (STLV-III), is closely related to HIV. It is similar to HIV in its growth and form and carries similar protein antigens. The antibodies of people with HIV binds with some of its viral antigens.

More than half the African green monkeys (AGM) raised in a closed colony at the Paul Ehrlich Institute in America have antibodies that bind with HIV, but are healthy. STLV-III$_{AGM}$ has been isolated from these animals and has killed both monkey and human T-lymphocytes in culture. STLV-III$_{AGM}$ has also been isolated from African patients with HIV and AIDS.

Although STLV-III$_{AGM}$ does not cause illness in African green monkeys, it induces an AIDS-like disease in Indian rhesus monkeys (macaques), many of which die with a wasting syndrome, immunological abnormalities, opportunistic infections and brain damage. Some, however, survive; their ability to survive is directly related to the strength of their antibody response.

Another strain of STLV – STLV-III$_{MAC}$ – is common in species of macaques (hence the designation), including the rhesus monkey, where it does not cause illness. Some African green monkeys have antibodies against STLV-III$_{MAC}$; these antibodies also bind with HIV isolated from people with AIDS.

Yet another retrovirus (SRV-I), quite different from STLV-III, has caused spontaneous outbreaks of Simian Acquired Immunodeficiency Disease (SAIDS) in macaque monkeys at the Californian Primate Research Center. Many of the clinical signs, immune defects and pathological changes of SAIDS resemble those of AIDS in people. In both, the central nervous system is a significant reservoir of latent virus. However, a vaccine prepared from inactivated SRV-I completely protects monkeys against the virulent disease.

Further research into all these viruses, into how they cause disease in monkeys, and, in particular, how some monkeys survive their infections, will lead to a better understanding of how HIV acts in people.

5 AIDS

The illness caused directly by HIV, which we have called the primary illness, is not AIDS. Many people recover from this primary illness, although they usually go on to develop AIDS within the next few years. We give the formal, medical, definition of AIDS later in this chapter, but first we describe some of the related conditions from which HIV-infected people may suffer as they progress towards AIDS. These include lymphadenopathy (swollen lymph glands); lesser AIDS; ARC (AIDS-Related Complex or Condition). These various conditions usually appear before AIDS is diagnosed, but they don't appear at any particular time, or necessarily in the order in which we describe them. Sometimes they don't appear at all: often they overlap and cannot clearly be separated. Not all the terms have a clear formal definition, nor are all used by all doctors.

Lymphadenopathy

Lymphadenopathy is swollen lymph nodes or glands (see page 41 for a diagram of the lymph system). Several viruses – including those which cause mumps and glandular fever – may result in forms of lymphadenopathy.

As we described in Chapter 4, HIV infects T4-lymphocytes and B-lymphocytes. The T4-lymphocytes are killed by the virus and T8-lymphocytes tend to increase in numbers to compensate. The virus also causes B-lymphocytes to proliferate. Most of the lymphocytes stay in the lymph nodes and spleen, which swell as the number of occupants increases. The lymph nodes may become two centimetres

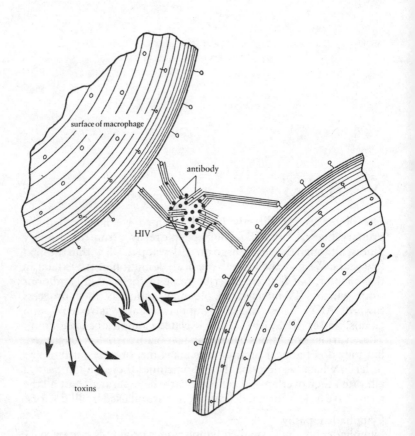

Specific antibody binds to HIV to form a 'complex', which sticks to macrophages in the lymph nodes, and which starts a chemical chain-reaction which produces toxins.

or more in diameter and are uncomfortable and occasionally painful. They can be felt under the jaw and in the neck, the armpits and the groin.

The antigens (chemicals foreign to the body) of HIV stick specifically to antibodies against HIV, and the antibodies then stick to macrophages in the lymph nodes. The combination of antigen and antibody causes a natural chemical in the blood to be changed into a toxin. The main action of this toxin is to kill bacteria, but it also causes the infected patient to feel unwell, and may result in fevers, chills and sweats. The combination of antigen and antibody is then absorbed by the macrophages. In such circumstances a bacterium would be digested and destroyed, but HIV remains alive inside macrophages, which may become reservoirs of latent virus.

Lymphadenopathy is accompanied by mild to severe immuno-deficiency: the patient becomes more susceptible to infections, and some viruses, fungi and bacteria which are normally harmless may cause diseases, such as mild pneumonia or thrush.

Lesser AIDS
The first strict definition of AIDS used throughout the world was drawn up by the Centers for Disease Control (CDC) in the USA. The definition did not include infection with HIV, and it did not embrace the wide range of clinical conditions and diseases that occur in people infected with HIV. The term 'lesser AIDS' was used in 1985 to describe immunodeficiency accompanied by oral thrush, *Herpes zoster* (which causes shingles), thrombocytopoenia (a reduction in the number of blood platelets), and tuberculosis, in the absence of any other causes of immunodeficiency and in the presence of HIV.

AIDS-Related Complex (ARC)
The term ARC originally applied to patients with many of the signs and symptoms of AIDS, but who did not meet the rigid criteria of the CDC. Now that infection with HIV, together with familiar signs and symptoms, is virtually diagnostic of AIDS, the term ARC is used to describe a pre-AIDS condition; a mild form that usually progresses to AIDS.

AIDS Dementia Complex (ADC)
HIV infects macrophages in the central nervous system as well as the rest of the body. The toxins which are formed around the macrophages (possibly formed by them) affect the brain, the spinal

cord and the nerves in several ways. Firstly, those nerve processes and pathways which cause the limbs to move may be disturbed, and may result in paralysis, loss of movement and uncontrolled movement. Secondly, the pathways in the brain which control a person's behaviour may be affected, and the person's manner may become different, unusual or unrecognisable. The changed behaviour ranges from withdrawal to violence. Finally, those nerve pathways may be affected which allow a person to recognise and understand their environment. As a result, the patient's understanding of reality, and their reponse to it, may change and become distorted. However, a similar form of mental confusion may also result from an overwhelming fear of AIDS in people who belong to a high-risk group, whether they are infected with HIV or not.

The various illnesses caused by damage to the brain, spinal cord and nerves are known as dementia. ADC may occur in HIV-infected people with no other signs or symptoms of AIDS, or at any other stage.

Acquired Immune Deficiency
The initials AIDS stand for Acquired Immune Deficiency Syndrome. A syndrome is a collection of signs and symptoms identified collectively as a single clinical entity or disease. The description of the signs and symptoms that form the diagnosis of AIDS is somewhat complex.

Immunodeficiency is a state in which the immune response of the body to antigens – chemicals foreign to the body – is reduced. B-lymphocytes, T-lymphocytes and macrophages, which make up the immune system, form part of a finely balanced system for defence against infection. The antigens of a virus are recognised by T-lymphocytes and macrophages, which present the information to the B-lymphocytes. The T-lymphocytes become activated, and they proliferate. Some of them attack the virus directly, or the cells in which the virus reproduces, and destroy them. Other T-lymphocytes help the B-lymphocytes to produce antibody that binds with antigens of the virus, and may either neutralise the virus or induce macrophages to consume it.

The deliberate elimination, or reduction in number, of any of these cells by means of drugs is known as immunosuppression. Immunosuppressive drugs may be given to a transplant patient, for example, to prevent a transplanted organ being rejected. By contrast, the elimination or reduction in number of any of these cells by disease is known as immunodeficiency. There are several forms of inherited or congenital immunodeficiency caused by the absence of certain genes. If a child is born with immunodeficiency, he or she usually dies within a few months or years because there is no immune mechanism to deal with infections. However, an acquired immunodeficiency may arise at any time during life. Most virus illnesses, such as influenza, result in a transient, acquired immuno-deficiency (lowered resistance), which can allow secondary bacterial or fungal infection to cause diseases like pneumonia or thrush, from which the body normally recovers. An infection with HIV results in an acquired immunodeficiency from which the body does not recover. The secondary infections (opportunistic infections) or cancers which result from the lowered resistance may overwhelm the body. It is these overwhelming opportunistic infections and cancers that constitute AIDS.

Opportunistic infections and cancers

An opportunistic infection is a microbe that does not usually cause disease in healthy people, but which takes the opportunity to do damage when the immune system is not working properly. Almost any opportunistic infection, and various cancers, can contribute to AIDS, but are diagnosed as AIDS only if they are unusually severe or long-lasting, and if there is an underlying immune deficiency caused by HIV infection, or if the underlying immune deficiency cannot be explained other than by HIV infection. Many of the infections and cancers also afflict people who are not infected with HIV but have an immune deficiency for some other reason – perhaps because they are being treated with certain drugs for cancer, or to combat transplant rejection. In such cases, the infections are not AIDS.

In the Western world the most common opportunistic infections of AIDS are *Pneumocystis carinii*, *Mycobacterium avium*, *Mycobacterium tuberculosis*, candida and cryptococcus.

Pneumocystis carinii is an organism which infects the lungs and causes a form of pneumonia. In the early stages of AIDS, this may appear as a dry cough which persists for several months. As the immune deficiency caused by HIV gets worse, the *P. carinii* spreads further and the pneumonia gets worse. Ninety-four per cent of patients who enter hospital and are diagnosed as having AIDS have *P. carinii* pneumonia.

Mycobacterium is a form of bacterium which causes tuberculosis. The common form, which damages the lungs and bones of people other than AIDS patients, is *M. tuberculosis*. In AIDS patients the disease progresses more rapidly and is more rapidly fatal than in other people. *M. avium* is an organism that causes tuberculosis in birds, and is an opportunistic infection in people with immune deficiency. Nearly half of the people diagnosed as having AIDS have a form of tuberculosis, often in addition to at least one other infection.

Candida albicans is a yeast, or fungus, which causes thrush, a white furry coating on the tongue or vagina. Healthy people are able to overcome thrush relatively easily, but in AIDS patients it persists for a long time and may spread to the gullet and lungs, where it causes considerable damage. Cryptococcus is an unusual bacterium which, in AIDS patients, usually causes meningitis and is very difficult to cure.

Other opportunistic infections include cytomegalovirus, which provokes ulcers, especially in the lungs; *Herpes simplex* virus, which normally causes cold sores or genital ulcers; *Varicella zoster* which normally causes shingles; and many other viral, bacterial, fungal and parasitic infections, for instance cryptosporidium and toxoplasma.

Of the cancers that affect people with AIDS, the most common is Kaposi's sarcoma. This is a form of skin cancer that has been particularly common among men – especially homosexual men – with AIDS, but is now slightly less common. Most cancers begin at a single site in the body and may then spread to secondary sites; they can spread especially rapidly when the patient is immunodeficient, as are AIDS patients. Kaposi's sarcoma may possibly be caused by a virus, perhaps cytomegalovirus, which can be transmitted sexually. In the USA 15 per cent of all male AIDS patients have developed Kaposi's sarcoma, and 95 per cent of the AIDS patients with Kaposi's sarcoma are homosexual or bisexual men. Only two per cent of women with AIDS have developed Kaposi's sarcoma. This form of cancer is very resistant to treatment; the average life expectancy of an AIDS patient with Kaposi's sarcoma is little more than six months.

Another form of Kaposi's sarcoma that is mild, affects older men and progresses slowly, has been endemic in Africa for many years, and has nothing to do with AIDS. This form is relatively easy to treat.

While Kaposi's sarcoma is the most common cancer of AIDS patients, a number of others affect them. These include lymphomas, especially in the lymphatic system and brain, Hodgkin's disease, and several unusual cancers, such as a cancer of the mouth and tongue caused by a papillomavirus. This virus, like cytomegalovirus, is present in most people, but causes no problems until the immune system becomes deficient.

The formal definition of AIDS

A case of AIDS is a person with one or more of the following 'indicator' diseases, depending on whether the person is known to be infected with HIV.

For a person not known to be infected with HIV, the indicator diseases are:

- Thrush of the throat, gullet or lungs;
- Cryptococcus or cryptosporidium with diarrhoea for more than one month;
- Cytomegalovirus in any organ other than the liver, spleen or lymph nodes;
- *Herpes simplex* virus causing one or more ulcers lasting for more than one month;
- Kaposi's sarcoma in a patient under 60;
- Lymphoma of the brain in a patient under 60;
- *Mycobacterium avium* or *Mycobacterium kansasi* (which cause forms of tuberculosis) spread throughout the body;
- Pneumonia caused by *Pneumocystis carinii;*
- Infection of the brain with organisms of the toxoplasma genus.

For a person known to be infected with HIV, the indicator diseases are the infections and cancers listed above, and any other cancer or severe infection.

Since 1987 the case definition of AIDS has placed great importance on whether or not a person is infected with HIV. The case definition given here is a summary of the detailed case definition given by the CDC; the full version is intended to be a standard definition so that the spread of AIDS can be monitored. Other syndromes, such as ARC and lymphadenopathy, are to be called 'HIV disease', but it will be several years before the old terms are discarded.

Dying from AIDS

Once AIDS has been diagnosed the patient may die fairly soon, though the time can vary from several weeks to several years. Most of those with an opportunistic infection die within two years of the diagnosis of AIDS; the average survival time is one year. Often the immune deficiency is so severe by the time of diagnosis that treatment is very difficult; between 22 and 30 per cent of patients die during the stay in hospital in which AIDS was diagnosed.

Recovering from AIDS

There is a little evidence that some AIDS patients may survive for a long time (more than six years), but it is too early to say whether any of them will recover. The statistical evidence suggests that the longer an AIDS patient survives, the better are his or her long-term chances of living.

AIDS in different groups

AIDS is not a clear-cut syndrome with symptoms common to all patients; the progress of the disease varies from person to person. It is possible, however, to see a pattern in some groups of patients.

Homosexual men

Many homosexual or bisexual men who get AIDS have *Pneumocystis carinii* pneumonia or Kaposi's sarcoma, or both. On average, men with both Kaposi's sarcoma and an opportunistic infection die about 14 months after diagnosis of AIDS.

Haemophiliacs

Many haemophiliacs become seropositive (that is, they develop antibodies against HIV) without symptoms of the primary illness caused by HIV. Fewer seropositive haemophiliacs than homosexuals go on to develop AIDS, and those that do take much longer to become ill. Some doctors have suggested that many seropositive haemophiliacs are not actually infected with HIV, but have been immunised by dead virus in their infusion factors. This is not to say that their immunity will protect them from a future infection with HIV, but it might explain why so few seropositive haemophiliacs develop AIDS, and it suggests that many will not now get the disease.

Children

Virtually all babies who are infected with HIV in the womb, at birth or by breast feeding, develop ARC or AIDS within two years. Most of them have recurrent infections, especially pneumonia and thrush, many get leukaemias and lymphomas, and a number have progressive brain damage. Babies are more susceptible to AIDS than adults or older children because their immune system is less well developed.

Africa

AIDS in African people in Africa seems to be somewhat different from AIDS in Europe and America. For instance, African people are exposed to a different range of opportunistic infections than

Europeans and Americans, such as malaria, tuberculosis, cryptococcus and a number of parasitic infections. *Pneumocystis carinii* pneumonia is rare in Africans, but common in European and American AIDS patients.

The most common manifestation of AIDS in Africans is chronic diarrhoea, which results in a dramatic and continuing loss of weight. For this reason AIDS has been called 'Slim' disease. For some years, until tests for HIV became available, Slim was regarded as a different disease.

Because of these differences and because tests for HIV are not commonplace, the World Health Organisation has adopted a special case definition of AIDS in Africa, namely a person with at least two of the major signs, in association with at least one of the minor signs, in the absence of other causes of immunosuppression than HIV infection.

The major signs are:

● weight loss greater than ten per cent of body weight;
● chronic diarrhoea for longer than one month;
● fever for longer than one month.

The minor signs are:

● persistent cough for longer than one month;
● general itching;
● recurrent shingles, or thrush in the mouth and throat;
● chronic and widespread *Herpes simplex*;
● lymphadenopathy.

The presence of aggressive and widespread Kaposi's sarcoma or cryptococcal meningitis is alone considered enough for diagnosing AIDS in Africans.

AIDS also has a longer incubation period in Africa than in Europe or America; it is transmitted mostly by heterosexual intercourse and perhaps by dirty hypodermic needles, insect bites and scarification (ritual skin scarring).

6 Blood and blood products

The blood is of such importance to our understanding of AIDS that we need to say something about its composition.

Blood is a fluid which is pumped by the heart along the arteries to the muscles, skin and other organs, and which flows back through the veins to the heart again.

Blood is a carrier: of oxygen from the lungs to the rest of the body, and of carbon dioxide from the rest of the body to the lungs; of digested food from the gut to the liver and the rest of the body, and of wastes from the body to the kidneys; of hormones from the places where they are made to the places where they are used. These are only some of its functions.

The liquid part of blood is plasma. When blood clots, fibres of fibrin separate out to form the clot; the clear, straw-coloured liquid left behind is serum. Many things are dissolved in the plasma, such as clotting Factors, antibodies, and many other proteins, carbohydrates, hormones and other chemicals. Suspended in the plasma are a number of cells, including red blood cells, white blood cells and platelets.

Whole blood
A normal adult person has about eight pints of blood. Loss of more than a pint or two is life-threatening; the restoration of the lost blood can save life.

The National Blood Transfusion Service in Great Britain, and various private, national and charitable blood banks in Europe,

North America and the rest of the world, collect blood from volunteer or paid donors, and store it until it is needed.

Whole, liquid blood is stored in glass bottles, or plastic bags, at 4°C to 10°C for up to 28 days. During liquid storage the quality of the blood deteriorates. After 28 days it is withdrawn and used for manufacturing blood products.

Blood can also be stored frozen, indefinitely: the plasma is separated from the cells, and frozen at about −40°C. The cells are treated with special preservatives, and then stored at the temperature of liquid nitrogen (−196°C). Before frozen blood can be transfused into a patient it must be thawed, washed and reconstituted. This can take several hours.

Clotting Factors
There are at least ten clotting Factors in normal blood. Clotting Factors are proteins which act in cascade: the first Factors in the cascade are activated by exposure to air and to chemicals released from platelets which have been damaged. Each molecule of activated Factor then activates many molecules of the next Factor in the cascade. Eventually a large number of molecules of the last Factors cause the release of fibrin from the blood. These fibres form the clot which plugs the hole and prevents the escape of more blood.

If any one of the Factors is missing, no clot can form, and the smallest cut or graze can result in a life-threatening loss of blood.

Patients with haemophilia have an inherited absence, or reduction, of one or more clotting Factors.

Some people lose blood through defective blood capillaries: this is von Willebrand's disease.

Plasma collected for the purpose, or out-of-date plasma, is pooled from many donors, and can be processed to obtain solutions rich in certain specific Factors.

Patients with haemophilia can administer enriched Factors to themselves at home. Someone with severe haemophilia may need to administer Factors regularly and often to avoid bleeding. In less severe conditions, the haemophiliac may adjust the dose and frequency of therapy as he, or rarely she, thinks appropriate.

Platelets
People with a deficiency of platelets suffer from thrombocytopoenia. This may result from a number of conditions, including autoimmune disease (in which the patient destroys his own platelets by producing antibodies against them) and cancers (in which one side-effect of the

drugs given to the patient causes the numbers of platelets to reduce). The blood of people with thrombocytopoenia does not clot normally. They may bleed from their skin, or mucous membranes, or gut. Bleeds may form a red or purple rash or more extensive bruising. There may be overt, life-threatening loss of blood.

Platelet concentrate, an enriched suspension of platelets in plasma, can be prepared from whole fresh blood. Platelet concentrates can be stored in the cold for only three to five days, or stored frozen indefinitely.

Platelets may be infused into patients with thrombocytopoenia to restore the normal concentration of platelets in blood, and to restore its ability to clot normally.

Gammaglobulins

Antibodies are large globular proteins dissolved in the blood plasma. Each antibody binds with a specific antigen: foreign organisms – such as bacteria, viruses, blood cells from someone else – all carry antigens to which specific antibodies bind. Proteins to which antibodies belong are classified as immunoglobulins or gammaglobulins.

Plasma donated for the purpose, or out-of-date plasma, is used to prepare a solution rich in gammaglobulins and deficient in the other components of blood. Non-specific gammaglobulins are administered to people who may have been infected with hepatitis.

Many transfusion centres select donors who have been exposed to particular antigens, such as those of tetanus toxin, or *Herpes zoster* virus; their plasma contains high concentrations of specific antibodies against those particular antigens (that is, they are hyperimmune), and gammaglobulins prepared from their plasma are rich in those antibodies. Such preparations are effective in protecting people against tetanus, or in curing the symptoms of shingles, caused by *Herpes zoster*.

Infusion and transfusion

Only whole blood is transfused. In the early days of blood transfusion, blood was taken directly from the artery of the donor and carried through a tube and needles directly into the vein of the recipient. Now that blood is collected and stored in banks, infusion would be a more appropriate word.

Other fluids, such as blood products, or saline solutions, or some drugs given in large volumes, are infused into the patient's vein.

Blood, blood products and HIV

If a blood donor is infected with HIV, the virus can pass through the processes of purification into several, but not all, of the blood products. Whole blood is not processed or purified, nor can it be heated to kill the virus. The cells derived from blood, such as red blood cells, white blood cells and platelets, are separated fairly crudely: the virus might be present in the fluid around the cells, even after they have been 'washed', and the virus might be present in some of the white blood cells such as T4-lymphocytes, B-lymphocytes and macrophages. Cells cannot be heated to kill the virus because this would also kill the cells. Plasma, clotting Factors and gamma-globulins are also separated from whole blood in a fairly crude way, and might contain the virus in solution.

Other blood products, such as albumin, are fairly pure and often dried for storage. No one has found HIV in these products and no one is known to have caught HIV from them.

There are several points about the risk of catching HIV from blood and blood products:

● people in high risk groups are asked not to give blood;
● all blood donors are tested for HIV. People who are infected are not allowed to give blood, and if they do their blood is not used. Some donors might be infected but not yet seropositive when they give blood: the Transfusion Service estimates that the chance of this happening is now better than one in five million;
● each unit of whole blood, red cells or platelets comes from only one person, but plasma and clotting Factors are separated from the blood of several thousand donors. An infected donor is very unlikely to have provided the single unit which a recipient receives, but another infected donor is very likely to be included in a pool of several thousand;
● blood products such as plasma and clotting Factors are pasteurised to kill any virus including HIV. Blood products are now regarded as free from infectious HIV.

7   The spread of AIDS from person to person

In 1986 Robert Gallo (one of the foremost AIDS researchers in the USA) pointed out that the study of the spread of AIDS was really the study of the spread of the Human Immunodeficiency Virus. HIV had been spreading from person to person long before it was 'discovered'. Its epidemiology (who it affected and how it was spread) was very difficult to study. It is now clear that this difficulty arose from the very long and variable incubation period of the virus.

We now know that HIV spreads from person to person in body fluids such as blood and semen. It has been isolated and cultured from peripheral blood (near the surface of the body), semen, saliva, tears and milk, and may be present in mucus and urine.

The virus is fragile and does not easily survive drying, heat or cold. It is *not* transmissible merely by contact – for example, shaking hands or hugging – and there are no recorded cases of transmission in the droplets from the nose or mouth resulting from sneezing or coughing.

The virus *is* transmitted in warm body fluids during sexual intercourse if either partner is infected; during pregnancy or childbirth if the mother is infected; during the transfusion of blood or blood products if any of the donors was infected; and during organ transplantation, skin grafting or artificial insemination if the donor was infected.

Transmission by homosexual men

Until recently, transmission between homosexual men has been the major means of dissemination of HIV across the United States and Europe.

During homosexual intercourse a man inserts his erect penis into another man's rectum through the anus. During insertion the skin in and around the anus may tear and bleed. If the recipient is infected with HIV, the virus may pass from the blood into the other's body through the mucous membrane of the penis and through cut and torn skin. However, surveys suggest that this happens less often than virus passing from the seminal fluid of an infected man into the body of the recipient through the mucous membrane, and cut and torn skin.

Fisting is the insertion of the hand or fist into the rectum through the anus. This stretches and generally tears the skin around the anus, and draws blood. Evidence suggests that the person who inserts his fist is more at risk (from AIDS) than the person into whom it is inserted.

It is clear that during intercourse the virus is transferred mostly in seminal fluid, but can be transferred by other fluids, especially blood. It is not clear whether there is a risk of the passive partner infecting the active one through faeces or rectal mucus.

Seminal fluid contains many proteins, some of which are immuno-suppressive – that is, they reduce the immune response to infection. A homosexual man who receives semen from other men becomes more susceptible to many virus infections, including Epstein–Barr virus, cytomegalovirus and HIV. These infections are more common in homosexual men than in other people. The human rectum has not evolved to cope with seminal fluid in the same way as the vagina: thus a woman who receives seminal fluid into her vagina does not become immunosuppressed in the same way.

Seminal fluid also contains many cells, including lymphocytes, macrophages and sperm. The T4-lymphocytes and macrophages are cells in which HIV can live and grow. Men who are infected with any virus have more lymphocytes and macrophages in their semen than men who are not infected. If they are also infected with HIV they pass more cells, and so more virus, into their partners along with the immunosuppressive proteins.

In the major US cities – such as Los Angeles, San Francisco and New York – some homosexual men form widely interconnecting networks of sexual encounters. In San Francisco, for example, during the 1970s and early 1980s, the public bathhouses became popular meeting places for homosexual men, who would have intercourse with many other men each day. The virus was spread rapidly and widely: it has been calculated that, between June 1982 and May 1984, 17 per cent of the homosexual men in the city became infected annually.

Among the homosexual men in San Francisco, the greatest risk of becoming infected with HIV comes from receptive (passive) anal intercourse with someone with AIDS whose symptoms have already appeared. Risk of infection, in decreasing order, comes also from receptive anal intercourse with any infected man, insertive fisting and receptive oral intercourse. Very few of the men who practised insertive (active) anal intercourse but not receptive anal intercourse have become infected.

The risk is also related to the number of partners. A study in San Francisco in 1985 classified men according to the number of their sexual partners, and compared them with heterosexual men.

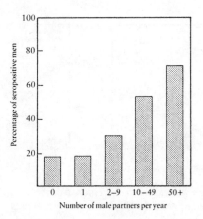

Research among homosexual and bisexual men in San Francisco in 1985 indicated a link between seropositivity and number of sexual partners.

The message here is very clear: the more male partners a man has, the more likely it is that some of them will be infected, and the more likely he is to catch HIV.

69

Between 1979 and 1983 the number of homosexual men with AIDS increased dramatically year by year. However, now (spring 1988), there is evidence of a marked reduction in the rate of acceleration of the AIDS epidemic among homosexual men around the world. Each year more homosexual men die of AIDS than in the previous year, but the rate of increase in numbers is not as great as it was. This phenomenon may have begun in the USA as early as 1983, and manifested itself as an actual reduction in other sexually transmitted diseases among homosexual men; it has been attributed to a fear of AIDS, causing homosexuals to change their practices.

A similar fear may have inhibited, or delayed, an AIDS epidemic among homosexual men in Sweden. During the 1970s the incidence of syphilis in homosexual men in Sweden had been increasing year by year. The first case of AIDS was reported at the end of 1982, and the public campaign against AIDS began in 1983. Since then, there have been major changes in homosexual behaviour, resulting in a sharp fall in syphilis and gonorrhoea among homosexual men. It is too early to know whether the campaign has halted the spread of HIV and AIDS.

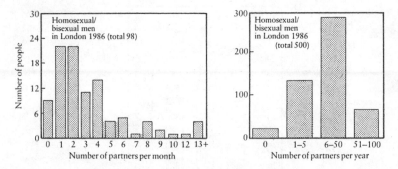

Homosexual and bisexual men tend to have more partners than heterosexual people. They form wide networks of sexual activity which spread HIV very quickly.

Transmission between the sexes

It is now clear that AIDS is not a disease of homosexual men alone: both men and women whose partners are infected with HIV or who have AIDS risk catching the virus and developing AIDS. Men and women whose partners are at risk (ie belong to any of the groups listed in Chapter 2) are also likely to catch the virus; women whose partners are bisexual are particularly at risk. Transfusions of blood donated by homosexual and bisexual men have also been shown to be a significant route of transfer, as have contaminated needles shared by drug addicts. Organ transplantation and artificial insemination from infected donors have contributed.

Heterosexual transmission, in both directions, appears to be the main way in which HIV spreads in Africa. Equal numbers of men and women are infected, and equal numbers develop AIDS. Many of the people who become AIDS patients have large numbers of sexual partners. Cases of AIDS and ARC form clusters linked by heterosexual contact networks. There is a high proportion of single women and female prostitutes among female AIDS patients, and a high rate of HIV infection among the spouses of AIDS and ARC patients.

During 1985, 1986 and 1987 the virus affected more women in the United States and Europe than ever before. Infected women then transmitted the virus to their male partners. During the four years to 1988 the virus has been spreading widely among heterosexual people.

It seems that, among female prostitutes, the spread of HIV is inhibited by the use of condoms (tests with high concentrations of virus at high pressures have shown that the virus particles will not pass through condoms of latex, lambskin or synthetic skin). In Zaire, for instance, more than 27 per cent of female prostitutes are estimated to be infected with HIV; in Kenya, the proportion is more than 59 per cent. The use of condoms by the clients of prostitutes in Zaire is associated with a lower rate of infection. In West Germany, many female prostitutes are licensed: because they regard the licence as valuable, they often insist on their clients using condoms; only about one per cent of them are infected with HIV. By contrast, many of the unlicensed prostitutes are drug addicts, and they rarely insist on the use of condoms; twenty per cent of the unlicensed prostitutes are infected with HIV.

The Centers for Disease Control (CDC), Atlanta, has been concerned about the number of AIDS patients who belong to no clearly identified risk group, that is, those who are not partners of infected people. 314 such patients were interviewed: 92 (out of the 314) appeared not to have been at risk of infection, but 37 patients (out of the 92) had had some other sexually transmitted disease: this suggested that they were relatively promiscuous although they had claimed not to be. Of the 92 patients, 49 men gave a history of sexual contact with a female prostitute. This suggests that sexual contact accounts for most of the cases of AIDS in people who appear not to be at risk.

By July 1987, 205 people in Britain and 1,500 people in the USA were known to have been infected with HIV by heterosexual contact. The risk of transmitting HIV in this way is between 20 per cent and 73 per cent: the range is wide because the ability both to infect and be infected varies widely from person to person and from time to time.

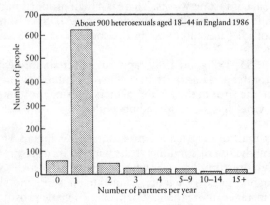

Heterosexual people tend to have fewer partners than homosexual men.

Transmission by blood

HIV has been transmitted by whole blood, packed red cells, platelet and white cell concentrates, and preparations of certain clotting Factors (see Chapter 6). There is no evidence that it has been transmitted by other blood products. How infectious a blood product may be is related to the numbers of infectious virus particles in it and to their capacity to multiply.

The virus has been spread by blood transfusion, but from early in 1986 two developments have dramatically reduced the risk to people needing blood and blood products in Europe and the USA.

Firstly, all blood donors in those areas are now tested for antibodies against HIV. Most transfusion centres ask people not to donate blood if they are infected or at risk of becoming infected. If they are found to be infected they are asked not to donate again, and their blood is withdrawn from the bank.

This has dramatically reduced the number of British blood donors with HIV antibody: the number fell to one sixth during 1987 in the North London region, where the chance of a recipient being transfused with infected blood is now (spring 1988) down to one in five million.

However, if the blood is donated during the virus incubation period, the test will give a negative result, and though the donor and the blood bank will be reassured, the recipient will be seriously at risk. There is evidence that a number of people who know they are at risk give blood in order to be tested for antibodies against HIV. Some blood banks in the USA offer 'Alternative Testing Sites' for people who want only to be tested for the virus, but who would otherwise give blood to obtain a result.

The second development reducing the risk to people, such as haemophiliacs, in need of blood products is that these are now pasteurised, and are therefore safe. Pasteurising involves heating the products to 56°C for 1 hour.

The Dutch Red Cross carried out experiments to measure the effects of pasteurising blood products for varying lengths of time. The samples were deliberately infected with a huge amount of HIV and then pasteurised. After eight hours, the infectiousness of the virus had been reduced by about 10,000 fold; after 72 hours it had been reduced, on average, by 100,000 fold (but by up to 10,000,000 fold). However, intensive testing of the samples showed that some virus capable of infecting always remained, albeit in very small amounts. They concluded that pasteurising should nevertheless prevent transmission of HIV.

In adults, the best estimate for the average incubation period of AIDS acquired by transfusion of infected blood is five years, although the most usual period is four years. In children infected by blood transfusion the average incubation period is five to six years, but the first symptoms generally appear between 9 and 13 months.

Before 1985

Until 1985, blood transfusion was a significant route of transmission of HIV. In West Germany, for instance, up to the end of 1985 HIV had been transmitted between 2,000 and 3,000 times by transfused blood: one in 500 units may have contained the virus. Or, again, of 18,406 cases of AIDS reported to the CDC in Atlanta in 1986, 284 (1.5 per cent) were related to blood transfusion. As a third example, 275 people were studied in the USA who had been infused with blood products from 61 donors who subsequently developed AIDS. After two years, 7 (out of 232 who were followed up) had developed AIDS; 130 (56 per cent) had antibodies against HIV – that is to say, they were infected.

It is estimated that altogether 45,000 recipients of blood in the USA may have been infected by the virus. By mid-1987 only 28 had developed AIDS, but more than 20,000 are expected to become seropositive, of whom more than 1,300 are expected to go on to get AIDS.

Haemophiliacs
Until 1985 haemophiliacs were a particularly vulnerable group. The likelihood of their seroconverting seems to have been related to their exposure to particular blood products. For instance, in an Australian study, 5 per cent of those haemophiliacs who suffered from Factor IX deficiency (Christmas Factor) seroconverted, while 25 per cent of those with von Willebrand's disease (loss of blood through defective blood capillaries) and 78 per cent with severe Factor VIII deficiency seroconverted.

Since the introduction of heat treatment of blood products in 1984, and the rigid exclusion of high-risk donors, there have been no seroconversions in Australia.

There are about 5,000 haemophiliacs in Britain; about 1,200 have antibodies against HIV and are probably infected. Since 1980 60 British haemophiliacs have developed AIDS and 45 of them have died. 18 wives have been infected, mostly by sexual intercourse with their husbands.

In the whole of the USA, up to 15 September 1986, 238 haemophiliac patients had developed AIDS (16 cases of AIDS per 1,000 haemophiliacs); in San Francisco, a very high proportion of haemophiliacs is seropositive, yet the incidence of AIDS is even lower (7.5 cases per 1,000 seropositives). This has raised the question of whether the virus in blood products is 'alive' at the time of infusion; however, live virus was cultured from 38 per cent (a high proportion) of tested seropositive haemophiliacs.

It is not clear why so few infected haemophiliacs develop AIDS – or why the incubation period is so long – but studies show that the probability of seroconversion in their group is related to low T4/T8 ratios in the patient (see Chapter 4), the number of vials of an infected batch which a patient uses, and the patient's total annual consumption of Factor VIII.

Transmission from mother to baby

It has now been proved that infected mothers transmit HIV to their foetuses; some experts have said that up to 95 per cent of infants born to infected mothers become infected – two thirds of them before birth, the rest at birth or from drinking infected human milk.

Others put the figure as low as 25 per cent in parts of Africa and 50 per cent among drug addicts in Edinburgh. It's now becoming clear that some infants do not develop antibodies for 20 months or more after birth, and they may have no symptoms during that time: it is then very difficult to associate infections with pregnancy, delivery or breastfeeding. Virtually all infected babies develop AIDS within two years.

It has been suggested (but not proven) that the risk of transmission of HIV during delivery may be reduced by delivery by Caesarean section. In an Italian study of 15 babies with HIV-infected mothers, all but one of the mothers was an intravenous drug abuser. Eight of the babies were born naturally: three of these became infected with HIV. Of the seven babies delivered by Caesarean section, none was infected.

In the USA up to the end of 1985, 231 children under 13 had developed AIDS – more than half of them in the second half of that year. Of these children 174 (75 per cent) had been infected from their mothers at or before birth; 19 per cent became infected from infusion of blood or blood products; in six per cent the source of infection was unknown.

Using a simple breakdown, the mothers of these 174 children were:

	per cent
Intravenous drug abusers	61
Haitian women	22
Women whose partners were at risk	15
Women who had received blood transfusions	1
Women who appeared not to be at risk	1

About 73 per cent of children who are infected by their mothers develop AIDS within their first year of life. The disease shows itself in several well-defined syndromes: inflammation of the lungs (39 per cent); miscellaneous infections (34 per cent); heart disease (32 per cent); brain damage (10 per cent); hepatitis (10 per cent) and calorie protein malnutrition (5 per cent). The children without symptoms of AIDS usually have immune defects and mild lymphadenopathy.

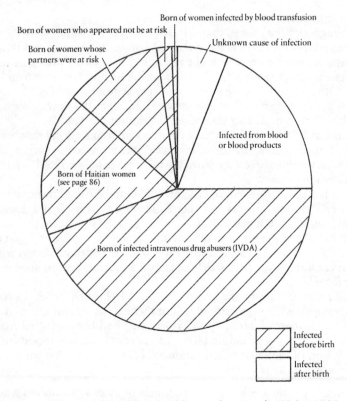

Sources of infection of the 231 US children under 13 with AIDS in 1985

The incubation period (the time between HIV infection and diagnosis of AIDS) is not clear, but it appears to range from less than 10 months to more than 21 months. In newborn infants, the average survival time after diagnosis is four months; in children infected some time after birth, eight months.

Diagnosis of HIV infection in babies is not always easy, since newborn babies may not produce enough antibodies for several days after birth to be detected, even longer if they are immuno-deficient, so a reliable diagnosis cannot be made until they are at least three months old, by which time they may already have developed ARC. Most doctors now assume that babies born of infected mothers are already infected.

Many doctors in many countries advise seropositive women to consider being sterilised, to avoid the possibility of pregnancy. They advise seropositive pregnant women to have abortions, because of the near-certainty of their bearing infected infants.

Transplants, skin grafts, donated sperm

Before 1985, recipients of organ transplants, skin grafts and donated sperm were at some risk from HIV infection, but during that year tests for infection became available, and by the end of

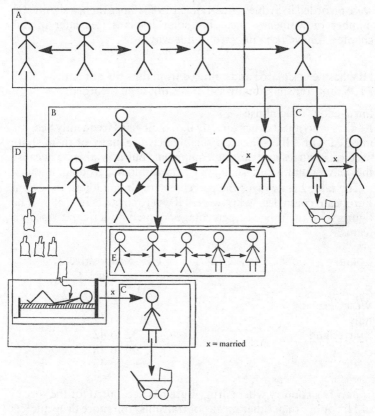

HIV spreads rapidly within groups of homosexual men (A) and less rapidly among sexually active groups of heterosexual people (B). It can be transmitted from mother to baby (C), from blood donor to the recipient of blood products (D) and between drug addicts who share needles (E).

1986 had been introduced into clinics throughout the developed world. Although the incidence of infection in these ways has been low, several cases of each kind have been reported. Curiously, each new way of infection seems to have been unexpected. The first case of transmission by a skin graft in the UK was as recently as February 1987; although testing of blood donors became routine in 1986, and tests were carried out on skin graft donors, it appears that doctors often did not wait for a result before grafting the skin.

The first cases of the transmission of HIV by artificial insemination were recorded in Sydney, Australia in 1983. Since then, a significant number of women – including some lesbians (see later in this chapter) – have been infected in this way.

Saliva
HIV has been isolated and cultured from the saliva of patients with AIDS, but transmission by saliva has not been recorded.

Intravenous drug abuse
Addicts who inject drugs directly into their veins frequently become infected with HIV. This is probably because many of them share needles, syringes and cutting equipment, but may also be because they have a number of sexual partners within the group of addicts.

The table below gives the percentage of drug addicts, in several European countries, who were HIV-seropositive in 1985. The figures give the range of percentages quoted by different research teams.

Country	HIV-seropositive (per cent)
England	1.5 to 6.4
West Germany	6
Italy	20.3 to 22.5
Switzerland	32 to 42
Austria	44 to 48
Spain	44 to 48

Italy is a country where drug abuse has accounted for the spread of HIV more than other means of transmission: more drug addicts are seropositive than any other group of people, including homosexual men. 52 per cent of intravenous drug abusers in Rome and 60 per cent in Milan were infected with HIV at the beginning of 1986. The frequency of HIV infection among drug addicts in Milan may lead to other infections and to death. Studies of female prostitutes around the world have all shown that those who inject drugs are much more likely to become infected than those who do not. It may be that the risk to drug-users is for some reason higher than the risk to those who have unprotected rectal or vaginal intercourse with men who are at risk, but this is difficult to judge: frequently, those prostitutes who do not use drugs insist on the use of condoms by their clients. Again, in Italy, the only seropositive prostitutes are those who inject drugs intravenously and those who do not use condoms. The same applies to female prostitutes in Los Angeles, New York and Florida, and West Germany where only one per cent of licensed prostitutes but 20 per cent of unlicensed prostitutes have HIV antibodies.

Close contact
HIV is not transmitted by close casual contact, as various studies have shown. For instance, in a special boarding school in France 24 severely haemophiliac children lived with 70 non-haemophiliacs. Over a three-year period half of the haemophiliacs became seropositive (from their infusion therapy), but none of the non-haemophiliacs.

A group of New York AIDS patients was studied over a number of years for the effects of casual contact with other members of their households, including children, siblings, parents and other relatives. Of 136 household contacts, only one became seropositive: the mother of the child had AIDS, and may have infected the child at, or before, birth.

In three other comparable studies, none of the household contacts of ARC or AIDS patients became seropositive during the study in question. In all these households, family members tended to share toothbrushes, towels, cutlery, crockery, drinking glasses, lavatories, razors, beds and combs, and there was a significant amount of hugging and kissing on the lips and cheeks; no incest was recorded, however.

Healthcare workers cannot avoid coming into close contact with AIDS patients, but the risk of their becoming infected is very low. Of 944 healthcare workers monitored by the CDC up till the end of 1986, only one became seropositive.

Lesbians
Lesbian women who have sex only with other women are at very little risk of AIDS, because little or no body fluid is transferred.

However, a lesbian Philippino appears to have caught HIV from her female lover. She denied ever having had sex with men, she did not take drugs and she had never received a blood transfusion. It is likely that the virus was carried in blood drawn during vigorous sexual stimulation, but it may have been transferred in vaginal secretions or, possibly, in saliva.

Those lesbians who also have sexual intercourse with men – especially bisexual or homosexual men – or who share drug-taking equipment with other people, are clearly at risk.

During the decade to 1982 it was fashionable in some large American cities for lesbians to be artificially inseminated with semen from homosexual men, and to bear their children. A number of these women, and their children, were infected with HIV in this way, and developed AIDS. Since 1986 all sperm donated to sperm banks is tested for HIV.

Rape
Anybody can be subjected to sexual intercourse by force. We have not found any records of women who have become infected with HIV as a result of a sexual assault of any kind. This is probably because the number of women raped is low (compared with the population) and the number of rapists infected with HIV is probably very low (compared with the population of men). In addition, it is difficult to pinpoint the date of infection. However, the possibility remains.

Aids in prisons
The incidence of HIV infection, and of AIDS, in prisons in the Eastern USA, in Britain and in Europe has increased dramatically since 1984. AIDS is probably spreading faster in men's prisons than in the general population. It seems to be spread mostly by homosexual intercourse, including rape, and to a lesser extent by sharing drug-taking equipment.

8 The spread of AIDS around the world

It's not entirely clear which route HIV has taken in its spread around the world. It first appeared in central Africa some time before 1979 but probably not before 1960; it was not recognised until 1983.

A likely suggestion is that a virus which causes AIDS in monkeys in Africa infected Africans, and then mutated to become HIV. The virus spread to the Caribbean, especially to Haiti on the island of Hispaniola, and then to the major cities of the United States, in particular, Los Angeles, New York and San Francisco. The first cases of AIDS were described and diagnosed in young homosexual men in Los Angeles in 1979.

HIV spread rapidly through the United States, and outwards into South America and Europe. The first British case of AIDS was diagnosed in Edinburgh in 1982. Meanwhile, the virus has been spreading rapidly within central Africa and outwards to the rest of the continent.

Africa

Many viruses closely or distantly related to HIV have been endemic in Africa for several decades – perhaps for centuries. Some of the viruses infect people, causing diseases ranging from the innocuous to the virulent; others infect animals – including monkeys – and, again, there is a range of diseases.

There have been suggestions that a monkey virus – such as STLV-

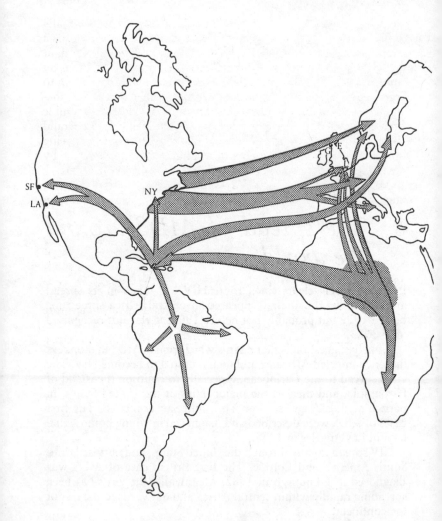

The spread of AIDS.

IV, which is very similar to both HTLV-IV and HIV (and especially similar to HIV2) – might have been transferred to people in a monkey bite, by eating monkey flesh or drinking monkey blood, or by bestiality. Many African tribes have used monkey blood as an aphrodisiac: 'To stimulate a man or a woman and induce them to intense sexual activity, male monkey blood (for a man) or she-monkey blood (for a woman) was directly inoculated in the pubic area and also into the thighs and back . . . ' This practice would inevitably introduce monkey viruses into the people who were being stimulated; the viruses would spread rapidly through the tribe by sexual intercourse, scarification and blood-brotherhood rituals.

Monkey viruses are not all dangerous to people (although some, such as Monkey B Virus, are deadly), but only a small mutation would have converted STLV-IV to HIV.

The ways AIDS has spread

Set against the wars, famines, chronic infections and poverty that central African countries were already confronting, AIDS was not seen as anything extraordinary; its occurrence and spread was not monitored until medical scientists in Europe and America became alerted. Even then, population sampling was difficult, inaccurate and expensive. Many African governments refused to co-operate: some denied that their country had AIDS; others saw it as a minor problem among many more important ones. Many scientific reports about AIDS in Africa are inadequate, and most are conflicting, so solid scientific evidence is lacking.

The spread of AIDS in Africa is unusual in the high proportion of people infected with HIV, and in the equal incidence in men and women. In general, single women, and men with many sexual partners, are most affected. Sexual intercourse seems to be the most common way the virus is transmitted. The very highest rates of seropositivity are in female prostitutes: the mobility of prostitutes across countries may have been an important factor in the spread of HIV and AIDS across Africa.

However, records held at sexually transmitted disease clinics in central Africa suggest that men may become infected from women less often than the incidence of HIV in the sexes would indicate, and that many men and women have been infected from re-used needles when blood was taken at the clinics. Some experts have put forward the idea that re-used needles – in hospitals, clinics and transfusion centres – might be the main way in which HIV is spread.

Another possible means of transmission is through bedbugs. There is evidence that HIV can survive in bedbugs for up to an hour. They are thought to regurgitate blood when starting to feed again after an interruption – such as changing host – and they are known to transmit hepatitis B. Other insects are known to transmit the retrovirus which causes equine infectious anaemia and bovine leukosis in a very similar way. Bedbug infestation is common in parts of Africa, where between 15 and 22 per cent of AIDS cases have been children. Most infected children live in underprivileged and low-income households, where they may share beds with adults. In these circumstances bedbugs may be a significant route of infection in children.

There is a very small likelihood that HIV can be spread in the malaria parasite, *Plasmodium falciparum*, which is transmitted by mosquitoes. The virus does not survive in mosquitoes themselves. In a study of 520 hospital (not necessarily AIDS) patients in Zaire, the incidence of HIV antibody correlated strongly with antibody against *Plasmodium falciparum*. The link is likely to be coincidental.

Symptoms and manifestations

Many apparently healthy Africans have activated T-lymphocytes (activation of T-lymphocytes appears to be the basic event regulating HIV propagation and subsequent death of the T-lymphocytes – see Chapter 4). Almost all of them have low-grade infections with parasites (such as malaria and schistosomes), fungi or tuberculosis. These subclinical infections may predispose Africans to easier infection by HIV as they may then develop into the opportunistic infections symptomatic of AIDS.

In Africa, as elsewhere, the disease includes lymphadenopathy associated with HIV infection. However, the opportunistic infections are different from those in Europe and America, probably because Africans are exposed to different opportunistic infections from Europeans or Americans. Some of the common opportunistic infections in African AIDS patients are *Herpes zoster* (which otherwise causes shingles), thrush (especially in the mouth), tuberculosis and meningitis. A syndrome of wasting, recurrent fever, diarrhoea and fatigue is also common, and is called Slim disease; its direct cause is not known, but it is AIDS. In Zambia and Uganda the aggressive form of Kaposi's sarcoma typical of AIDS is common.

In Africa generally, clinical record-keeping has been a low priority. It is not clear, therefore, whether AIDS is new to the continent, or whether it has been present for many decades. Local doctors find it hard to imagine that infections as florid as oral thrush would have been overlooked consistently for decades; they have therefore decided that it is recent.

The routes HIV took

The first cases of AIDS in Africans were confirmed in Europe in 1981 and in Africa in 1983. The way the disease emerged is unclear because of variations in surveillance and reporting. One suggestion is that HIV may have infected some people in Zaire even before 1960: a sample of blood taken in 1959 from a person in Zaire, and tested in 1986, had traces of antibody against HIV. However, we know that tests for antibody could not, in 1986, distinguish between HIV and STLV-IV, and we know that many central Africans have antibodies against STLV-IV. Calculations of the rate of spread of HIV in Zaire suggest that the infection may have started in the central African cities as long ago as 1940. But these are speculations and calculations, not clinical observations.

The AIDS epidemic in Zaire's capital, Kinshasa, and in Kigali in Rwanda began in 1980 as cases of cryptococcal meningitis. The epidemic itself started in Zaire in 1982, but was not recognised until 1983, as aggressive Kaposi's sarcoma. Early in 1983, doctors in

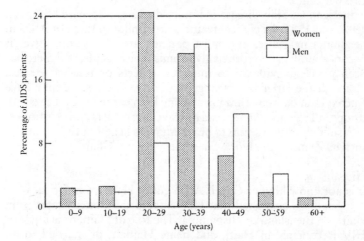

The first 500 cases of AIDS in Kinshasa. Heterosexually active people between 20 and 50 were in the majority.

Brussels and Paris reported an AIDS-like illness among patients from Zaire and Rwanda whose lifestyle appeared not to expose them to risk. At the same time it appeared in southern Uganda as both aggressive Kaposi's sarcoma and Slim disease. An epidemic of Slim disease began in Tanzania in 1984. (Recently, however, it has been suggested that the antibodies in these seropositive Africans might have been antibodies against other retroviruses, such as HTLV-I, HTLV-II and STLV, rather than against HIV.)

Clinical records suggest that in Rwanda and Zambia, AIDS affects the affluent, but that the opposite is true in Zaire and Uganda. It is possible, therefore, that AIDS has been endemic for a long time among the poor of Africa, and spread to the affluent around 1980. There has been a tenfold increase in seropositivity in the population of Zaire in the past ten years.

HIV appears to have arrived in Kenya in about 1980 or 1981 – possibly five years after it arrived in the United States. The prevalence of antibodies in Kenyan prostitutes rose from 4 per cent in 1981 to 59 per cent in 1985. 95 per cent of the prostitutes in Kenya appear to originate from Tanzania or Uganda. Among men with genital ulcers (a condition which suggests promiscuity), none had HIV in 1980, while 14 per cent had antibody in 1984. The prevalence of antibody in pregnant women was zero in 1981, and two per cent in 1985.

In Uganda, Slim disease is reported to have appeared between 1982 and 1985. Its clinical features are similar to those of AIDS in neighbouring Zaire, and most patients are HIV-seropositive. It occurs mainly in heterosexually promiscuous people, and there has been no clear evidence to implicate insects or re-used needles, although the latter is a strong possibility. The disease may have entered Uganda from Tanzania, having been carried in by Tanzanian troops in 1980 and then spread by travelling traders and prostitutes.

A similar pattern seems to be emerging in neighbouring countries such as Zambia, the Ivory Coast, Senegal and Ghana.

Hispaniola

It is not know how or even if AIDS got to Haiti from Africa.

It has been suggested that HIV entered the United States from Haiti, on the island of Hispaniola. The role of Haitians is unclear. HIV is endemic in Haiti, and being Haitian, or married to an Haitian, or born of Haitian parents, is regarded by the Centers for Disease Control in Atlanta as a risk factor for AIDS on the same level as being a homosexual man with many partners or a drug addict.

It has been suggested that homosexual men from Los Angeles, San Francisco and New York – American cities well known as centres of male homosexual networks – may have visited Haiti as tourists during the 1970s and become clients of inexpensive male prostitutes. They then carried the virus back to their local networks. Two factors may have made this transfer easy: during the 1960s and 1970s air travel and tourism became easy and cheap; and public acknowledgement of homosexuality was followed by a period of extroversion among male homosexuals. Transmission of HIV among Haitians living in the United States is almost entirely by heterosexual intercourse.

HIV was not transferred over the border into the Dominican Republic on the eastern side of the island. Haitian workers cross into the Dominican Republic to cut cane in season, and then return home. Although a high proportion of these healthy Haitian workers have HIV, but not AIDS, only a small proportion of Dominican male homosexuals have HIV. Dominican drug addicts are not infected, possibly because the supply of drugs is restricted, and they are able to buy new needles quite freely from the pharmacies.

USA

In the USA, the first AIDS patients were recognised in Los Angeles in 1979. Within months the syndrome was recognised in a number of homosexual men in Los Angeles, San Francisco and New York. The virus, and syndrome, spread rapidly through the male homosexual and bisexual networks of these three US cities. For single men aged between 25 and 44 in Manhattan and San Francisco, AIDS was the leading cause of mortality in 1984.

Infection with HIV is much more common in high risk groups of people than is AIDS.

A total of 135,000 cases of AIDS arising from blood transfusions is expected in the USA by 1991 – all of them infected before 1986. These estimates take into account neither new infections after 1985 nor very long incubation periods. They are therefore the smallest numbers to be expected.

New York City accounts for half the cases of childhood AIDS in the US, and for most of the cases of maternally transmitted disease. 94 out of 103 children with AIDS probably acquired it from an infected mother, at or before birth. It is calculated that 500 infected babies are born each year in the US.

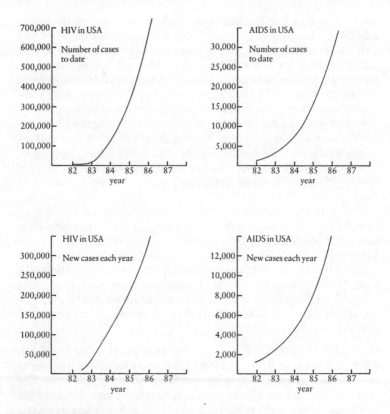

In the USA the number of new cases of AIDS reported each year is far greater than the number in the year before. The numbers of people infected with HIV is an estimate; the CDC believes that the quoted figures are underestimated.

AIDS is spreading rapidly through the prisons of the United States. Some penal institutions have recorded a doubling of the number of cases each year, and AIDS has now been diagnosed in women's prisons. A very small number of prisons in the mid-Atlantic seaboard of the US accounts for almost 70 per cent of AIDS in US prisoners.

Since the middle of 1986 there has been a marked fall in the incidence of sexually transmitted diseases, other than AIDS, in

American homosexual men. This fall has been attributed to a change in sexual behaviour induced by a fear of AIDS.

At the same time, there has been a reduction in the rate of acceleration of the AIDS epidemic in the USA. At the end of 1987 the epidemic was still accelerating, but not as rapidly as it had been at the end of 1985.

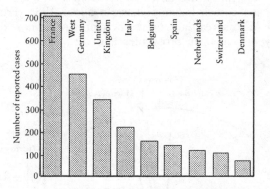

The number of cases of AIDS in nine European countries up to March 1986

Italy

In Italy, intravenous drug abusers are the main risk group for HIV infection – even more than male homosexuals. It seems that HIV reached Milan first and then spread to other Italian cities. The first HIV-seropositive blood sample was taken in February 1979. The numbers increased sharply (see Chapter 7). AIDS was first diagnosed in Italy in 1982, three years after the first diagnoses in the USA.

It has not been possible to separate transmission by drug abuse from transmission by prostitutes. A study of 29 Italian female prostitutes showed that the clients of those who were not drug users always used condoms, while the clients of those who were intravenous drug users rarely did so. 58 per cent of the prostitutes who were drug users were seropositive: none of those who did not use drugs was.

In Italy, there is an unusually high proportion of children with AIDS, most of them born of drug-addicted mothers.

Switzerland
Switzerland has one of the highest AIDS death rates in Europe, possibly because it appeared earlier in Switzerland than elsewhere.

HIV antibody was detected in drug abusers in Berne in 1982: in 1984, 42 per cent of Swiss drug abusers had antibody.

Great Britain
HIV is spreading in Europe, and in the United Kingdom, in much the same way that it has in the United States. HIV antibody first appeared in Scottish haemophiliacs in about 1981. From 1982 HIV and AIDS spread among the networks of homosexual men, especially among male prostitutes and their clients.

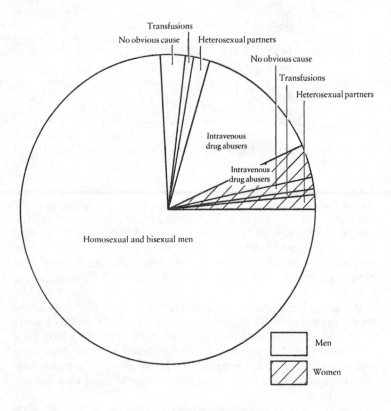

The distribution of AIDS in the UK

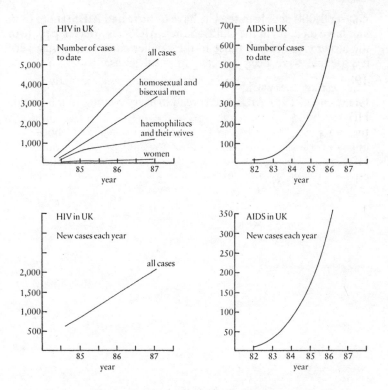

There are fewer cases of AIDS in the UK than in the USA (see the graph on page 88) but the numbers are increasing at the same rate. The Public Health Laboratory Service believes that the numbers of HIV-positive people are underestimated: there may be as many as 40,000 in the UK.

The virus then spread into the network of drug addicts who share needles. Healthcare workers are convinced that many more drug addicts, possibly ten times as many, are infected with HIV than are reported in the national statistics.

The virus is now (1988) being spread by sexual intercourse between men and women, and by analogy with the USA we can expect the number of cases of AIDS caused in this way to increase rapidly in the next few years. The number of homosexual men and drug addicts with HIV has increased dramatically since 1982.

91

Over 1,000 people in the UK have or have had AIDS: more than half have died. As in the United States, AIDS has affected people in the larger cities before those in the smaller cities and towns: very few people have been affected in rural areas.

The rest of the world
By the end of 1987 AIDS had spread to every country in the world.

9 The HIV test and beyond

Considering the test

If you are worried that you might be carrying HIV you can take a blood test called the HIV antibody test. This will show whether you have developed antibodies against HIV – that is, if you have been infected with the virus. It will not tell you if you will go on to develop AIDS – no test can tell you that.

Before you decide to have this blood test, consider it very carefully. A negative result may not end all your worries. Whether your result is positive or negative you may find that people you have told about the test change their attitude towards you. On the other hand, if you *are* infected with HIV, having the test will bring you into contact with help and advice on how to cope before, if and when you develop AIDS.

If you want advice on whether or not to have the test, you don't need to ask your friends – there are AIDS specialists and counsellors whose job is to give impartial and helpful advice; see Chapter 12. In fact, you would be wise to tell as few people as you need to that you are considering being tested because regardless of the result you may still lay yourself open to prejudice.

Where to go for the test

You can take the HIV antibody test at:

- any STD (Sexually Transmitted Disease) or GUM (Genito-Urinary Medicine) clinic
- your doctor's surgery

● a private clinic
● your Haemophilia Centre (if you or your partner is haemophiliac).

The test is free (other than at a private clinic) and confidential. You may feel more comfortable and anonymous if you take the test at an STD or GUM clinic rather than going to your own doctor. Your doctor will not be told the result unless he or she carries out the test, although they will be able to give you better care if you do offer the information. To find your nearest clinic, look in the telephone directory under Clinics, Venereal Diseases, VD, Sexually Transmitted Diseases or STD clinics; many directories list such clinics near the front. It's best to telephone before you go along, as some clinics prefer you to make an appointment.

Even if you have had earlier counselling, you should be offered further counselling before the test itself. A small sample of blood is then taken from a vein in your arm, a process which is not painful but may be slightly uncomfortable. You will have to wait for a short period (which may be a matter of days or up to about three weeks) to hear the result and find out whether or not antibodies to HIV are present in your blood.

What to do while you're waiting for the results

If you think you are infected with HIV, then anyone who has sexual intercourse or shares needles with you risks becoming infected too. It would be best to refrain from sex altogether until you are quite sure you are not infected. If you have to take drugs intravenously, keep your equipment clean and don't share it. In other words, behave as if you were infected with HIV and able to spread it until you know that you are not.

The results of the blood test

Your doctor or counsellor should tell you the result in person, and give you the opportunity to discuss the consequences there and then. You may like to bring your partner or a friend to hear the outcome of the test with you.

A *positive result* means that HIV has at some time entered your body and caused a reaction, that is, caused it to create antibodies. A person with antibody against HIV is said to be HIV-seropositive. Even if you are HIV-seropositive you may not have AIDS and may not get it, at least for some time. The doctor or counsellor should put you in touch with an appropriate agency to give you further support and advice.

A *negative result* means that you are probably not infected but it is important not to regard it as definitive. This is because it can take three months for your body to produce enough antibodies to be detected after infection with HIV and you may have been infected during the three months immediately before the test. During this time the test will be negative but you might be infected – and infectious. However, if you take a second test three months later and avoid sexual intercourse and receiving blood in the intervening period, you can infer from a second negative result that you are not infected.

The tests
The most common blood test for antibodies against HIV is known as ELISA (enzyme-linked immunosorbent assay). The test comes in several forms but basically involves a procedure where a blood sample taken from the person to be tested is allowed to clot. The serum is removed from the clot and added to a small test tube which is ready-coated with HIV antigen; any HIV antibody in the serum will bind with the antigen. The test tube is then treated with a preparation that includes a colour-change enzyme. When a chemical colour is added to the test tube, a change of colour indicates the presence of HIV antibody – a positive result; conversely, if the test tube stays the same colour, no HIV antibody is present – a negative result.

A number of things in the blood may interfere with the ELISA test, making it appear positive when it is not. Falsely negative results are rare, but falsely positive results occur in up to nine per cent of tests. For instance, plasma sometimes appears seropositive even when HIV antibodies are not present; blood which has not clotted fully (such as that from haemophiliacs) may show up as positive when it isn't; and infections from some parasites may also cause a positive result.

No one is told of a positive result until it has been confirmed by a repeat test.

A more sensitive test than ELISA, and one which can detect lower concentrations of HIV antibody and thus give a result much sooner (five or six weeks) after infection, is the Western Blot. This is a method of breaking down a blood sample into proteins by passing an electric current through it. Subsequent transfer of the proteins to a strip of treated paper, followed by a colouring process similar to that involved in ELISA, will show up the presence of any HIV. The

95

disadvantage of this test is that it is too complex and expensive for general screening.

A third test involves separating T-lymphocytes from a sample of blood and adding them to other T-lymphocytes which have been modified to grow in culture. If HIV is present in the blood sample, it can sometimes be cultured too. Unlike the general screening tests, the result is often falsely negative; this could mean that you have not been in contact with HIV, but it could also mean that you are infected but there was no active HIV in the sample or that no infected T-lymphocytes were present.

A fourth test involves the identification of reverse transcriptase (RT), an enzyme which enables a virus to incorporate its genes into a cell. The presence of RT in the blood of an immunodeficient person will confirm HIV infection. This test is expensive, time-consuming and requires a great deal of skill to perform.

Yet another test for HIV is the identification of HIV nucleic acid in the blood sample, but this test may not pick up all strains of HIV.

Tests are being developed to detect HIV antibody in saliva, but for the time being most tests require a sample of blood.

With all these tests it is important to remember that HIV takes some time to become detectable, so a negative result should always be followed up by a repeat test three months later.

CASE HISTORY

A 55-year-old woman with no symptoms was tested for HIV antibodies by an ELISA test, and found to be positive. The result was confirmed by a Western Blot.

Her husband had been transfused with three units of blood two years before. He was given every test for HIV, and found to have no antibodies against it.

Another sample of the woman's blood was put through a different set of tests, which turned out to be negative.

All the tests were analysed. The two with which the woman was first tested contained a particular protein against which she had antibodies. This protein was not relevant to HIV infection. These two results were 'false positives'.

Both the woman and her husband suffered considerable anxiety for several weeks.

A negative result?

If both your first and second results are negative, you should not forget in your relief that you may still encounter prejudice from anyone you may have told that you were undergoing tests. You may also feel discriminated against if you want to apply for a pension policy, a mortgage or any other form of insurance cover.

The Association of British Insurers has suggested to its members that anyone applying for life insurance should answer a question about AIDS – whether advice about or treatment for AIDS has been sought or a blood test taken. Anyone infected with HIV will be refused cover.

Any young single man applying for life insurance is regarded as a 'cause for inquiry' by insurance companies. Even if you answer 'no' to the question about AIDS, you are likely to get cover but at a higher rate than if you are a young married man. If you answer 'yes' to having had the blood test, or having sought advice or treatment, you may find it difficult to get cover, even if you are not infected.

Some insurance companies ask single men seeking life insurance to complete a separate questionnaire on AIDS. You are not asked specifically if you are homosexual, but if there is any indication of a relationship with another man, you are charged an extra premium, because of the AIDS risk. Insurance companies may ask doctors for information on applicants, and if your GP knows you have had a test he or she will be bound to disclose it.

If you possess insurance already the small print in your policy may oblige you to state any change in your circumstances; this could include taking the blood test – read the small print on your own insurance form to check whether this is essential.

A positive result?

Arrange to be tested again, with a different form of test. Several are available, from several manufacturers. Sometimes a single test can be falsely positive: several different tests are unlikely all to be falsely positive.

First, find someone with whom you can talk. Be sure that this person will be sympathetic and helpful. You may prefer to talk to someone you already know, such as a close friend, a parent or relation, your priest or doctor. Arrange a meeting where you will not be disturbed: the conversation may be emotional and long. You are asking your friend for a sympathetic ear, a shoulder on which to cry and perhaps for practical advice. If your friend reacts badly and is not sympathetic, don't pursue the conversation.

97

You may prefer to talk to a stranger, either directly or anonymously. You may find it most helpful to talk to someone in a similar situation to yourself, for instance a fellow haemophiliac or another homosexual. From the lists in Chapter 12 you can assess the sort of counselling you might prefer: if you don't like it, talk to someone else, but if you find yourself running from one person to another, seek medical help.

You may prefer to talk to an expert. If you took the test at a Sexually Transmitted Disease (STD) clinic or a Genito-Urinary Medicine (GUM) clinic, you will have been able to talk to a counsellor immediately. If you didn't discuss it at the time you can make an appointment to go back. These counsellors are specially trained to help people with HIV or AIDS. If they don't know the answers to your questions they will know where to find them.

If your own doctor arranged for your test, he or she will arrange for you to talk to a counsellor.

How will you feel?
Emotionally, it depends on you. You may have a positive, optimistic approach to life, enabling you to make the best of all situations. On the other hand, some people become anxious and frightened, and want immediate help and advice.

A few people become irrational, angry and abusive: they want to punish others – especially those in authority – for what has happened to them. If you are feeling like this or if you resent people's kindness or their prejudice, and want to hurt them, consider going to your doctor to explain how you feel. This kind of anger may for some people be the first sign of dementia. If your own doctor is not helpful, ask one of the organisations listed in Chapter 12 for the name of a doctor who will help.

Because you are infected with HIV you may be physically ill, with something like influenza or glandular fever. You may have swollen glands: you may even have an infection which gives you a cough, diarrhoea or thrush. If so, you should get advice, preferably from your own doctor, but if you can't be sure that he or she will be sympathetic, go back to the clinic or to another doctor.

If you are addicted to drugs you may be very ill. See a doctor urgently, and ask to be referred to a drug dependency clinic.

Whom should you tell?
You must tell any insurance companies who are providing you with life assurance: they are not obliged to honour your policies if you withhold the information that you are HIV-positive.

Otherwise you need not tell anyone, but you may find that it helps you emotionally if you do.

You may feel that you have a strong obligation to tell your spouse or lover if you haven't already confided in him or her. You may have to face a whole gamut of emotions and may in any case find it helpful to receive some counselling together.

If you have been faithful to the person with whom you have sex (and there can be no other source of infection), then you must have been infected by your partner – who may not know. Your partner may not thank you for the information, but the information ought to be passed back to the person who was the source of infection and so prevent its further spread.

If you've recently had sex with more than one person, you may not know who has infected you, or whom you have infected. It's just possible that the whole group with whom you associate is infected, but it's more likely that some people are, and some people aren't yet. By speaking out, you could break the chain of infection (see the diagram on page 77). Again, you may have to face a range of reactions, from abuse to sympathetic concern.

If you have donated blood, plasma, semen or milk within the last four months, you should tell the bank that you are now infected with HIV. The donation you gave may have live virus in it, and may infect someone else – but it may not have antibodies, and test results may have been negative at that time. It is very important that the bank should track down all the people who received your donation. At the same time, they will maintain your confidentiality.

If you are a haemophiliac you will probably have discussed with your family the chances of your becoming infected. They may know that you have been tested, and they will certainly want to know the result. They will probably want to help and comfort you, but they will also want to know how they can avoid becoming infected themselves – see later in this chapter.

You would be advised to tell the people who provide you (and possibly your family) with health care. Your doctor and dentist should be told so that they can avoid infecting themselves and their other patients. They will want to watch for signs of your illness getting worse, so that they can treat you early rather than late. Reputable practitioners will anyway sterilise all their equipment and take other precautionary measures, such as wearing surgical gloves. If your dentist refuses to treat you, the clinic where you took your blood test will help you find another one.

You may also consider it appropriate to tell anyone who looks after you or your relations in your home, such as the district nurse and midwife, the welfare workers, even your home help. Again, see later in this chapter for more information on protecting them from infection with HIV.

You are under no obligation to tell your employer or colleagues about your infection. Fear of dismissal should not deter you from telling them, though, if you decide that this would be best in your situation, because if you were dismissed you could make an application to an industrial tribunal. (Employment legislation gives this right to an employee who has been employed for two years or more – one year for those who began work before 1 June 1985 in firms employing more than 20 people; see Chapter 12 under Employment for where to get further advice.) However, in the past some people have not felt able to go through with such a tribunal because of the attendant publicity. Anyway, employers will more likely appreciate advice from you about how they can protect themselves and other staff. For instance, some hospitals and clinics are now providing employers with special packs containing plastic gloves, aprons and bags to add to their ordinary first aid supplies.

If you decide not to tell your employer and workmates, you can still suggest improvements in safety practices and first aid procedures. You may take positive steps to reduce and prevent the spread of infection, without causing panic. Be warned, though, that you cannot expect to protect others if you have an accident at work and they do not know that you are infectious.

Your sex life
If you are infected with HIV you should not have sexual intercourse with someone who is not infected. Sex with someone who *is* infected is also highly inadvisable, because you may lay yourself open to any number of other venereal diseases, such as syphilis or gonorrhea, some of which could become opportunistic infections that could trigger AIDS.

Discuss with your partner ways of adapting your sex life so that you can enjoy one another and remove the risk of transferring infection. If either you or your partner thinks that sex is too risky, you may agree to stop sharing it.

You can reduce the risk, but not eliminate it, by using a condom correctly. Read the instructions carefully. Squeeze the air from the tip of the condom before fitting it. It must cover the erect penis before any fluid from one person touches the other, and before approach or entry. After ejaculation the condom should be held firmly in place on the penis while it is withdrawn. The condom should be removed, tied and discarded safely in a sealed bag in the bin – not down the lavatory as condoms are a nuisance in the sewerage system.

Use a good quality product – not all contraceptive condoms are equally protective, and some break more readily in use. Extra-strong condoms are specially made for anal intercourse, but may also break. Generally speaking, the thicker the condom, the stronger it will be.

Many couples find pleasure in hugging, kissing and caressing, culminating in mutual masturbation. Avoid contact with seminal fluid, blood, vaginal fluid and milk. Moderate biting or vigorous rubbing – especially of the lips, penis, vulva, vagina and anus – can draw blood. The presence of a hangnail on the finger, or a cut or scratch on the hand, or a bitten lip, can result in an exchange of blood and of HIV. Cuts or sores on the hands and fingers can be protected with surgical gloves. Men can wear a condom for collecting infected seminal fluid, which can then be discarded safely. The vulva and vagina may safely be stimulated with a penile toy or dildo, but this should not be shared.

Household hygiene
The risk of infecting your friends and family – other than your lover – is very small; but you can reduce the risks even further by improving your levels of household hygiene.

Ordinary bleach, diluted one part bleach to nine parts water, kills HIV. Use it for cleaning up spilt blood, vomit, semen and other body fluids. Bleach should also be used to clean lavatories, baths, washbasins and sinks. Rubber gloves should be worn for such jobs.

Clean cutlery, crockery and razor blades with detergent and water hot enough to need to wear gloves. Rinse them in similarly hot water, and allow to dry without using a drying-up cloth or tea towel.

Don't let other people use your comb, razor or toothbrush, and don't use theirs. Clean these things as soon as possible after use. Clean out the hairs from your electric razor into the lavatory pan and flush them away: clean the razor head by running it in methylated spirit. Be meticulous about washing your own underwear – the hot cycle on the washing machine will kill any virus.

Don't pick at scabs. Clean all cuts, bruises, scratches, hangnails –

anything which bleeds or oozes fluid, no matter how trivial – with antiseptic, and cover with a waterproof dressing. When you remove it, discard the dressing carefully in a knotted plastic bag, not directly into the pedal bin. Toothpicks and dental floss should be similarly treated. Persuade other members of your household to do the same.

Menstrual blood also carries HIV and this contaminates tampons, sanitary towels and liners. Tampons may be flushed down the lavatory, which should then be cleaned with household bleach; dispose of towels and liners in knotted plastic bags, or burn them. Stained underclothes and linen should be soaked promptly in salt or biological detergent, and then washed with very hot water and detergent. Flush the salt or biological detergent away with bleach.

People who are HIV-positive are at much higher risk from infections than others. Some germs which would not hurt a healthy person could trigger AIDS in an HIV-positive one, so it is important, for instance, to thaw frozen food properly and to cook it thoroughly; wash your hands after handling pets and litter trays; and avoid contact with anyone who has a cold or a stomach upset.

Being positive

When you have got over the initial shock of a positive result, you would be wise to draw up a plan of action for yourself. Remember that being HIV-positive does not necessarily mean that you will go on to develop AIDS, but you should insist on giving yourself every chance of health.

Pamper yourself with long baths, lie-ins, massages. Improve the quality of your life by exercise, and improve your diet. Although we have found no scientific evidence that exercise and a good diet delay the onset of AIDS or may indeed prevent it altogether, it is worth pursuing, not least because it will make you feel good and will occupy you productively.

Create a support network of family and friends, and develop interests that you have always intended to pursue. Being active will help to reduce stress and keep anxiety and depression at bay.

You might consider giving time to a charity or other voluntary group, particularly one concerned with AIDS, if you feel able to offer support to others who may be more ill than you are.

If you have a faith, then prayer and greater commitment of time and effort to your religious group will ease your mind, and give a more positive meaning to your life.

Addictions

If you are addicted to drugs you should ask for expert help. Drug addiction and drugs weaken your resistance to disease: the combination of drugs and HIV infection could kill you quite quickly. Go to your doctor, or a clinic, or your hospital accident department.

If you inject drugs, and share your equipment with other people, go to a chemist or a clinic for new needles and syringes – keep them for your own use – and ask for expert medical help to cure your addiction.

If you are an alcoholic, or just drink too much, you risk having an accident or a fight or having casual sex and infecting other people with your blood. Whether you are an alcoholic or not, get help (such as from Alcoholics Anonymous) to stop you drinking altogether.

Pregnancy

It has been suggested that pregnant women infected with HIV develop AIDS more quickly than women who are not pregnant, but we have found little scientific evidence to support this suggestion.

However, if you are infected with HIV it is very likely that your baby will become infected during your pregnancy, or during delivery or by breast-feeding. A baby's resistance to disease is much less than that of an adult: babies who are born with HIV develop AIDS within a few months, and die within a year or two.

If you have HIV and are pregnant you should very seriously consider having your pregnancy terminated. Talk to your doctor, and visit your ante-natal clinic as soon as you can.

Many doctors have suggested that women infected with HIV should be sterilised, so that there is no chance of their bearing a child with HIV or AIDS. But sterilisation is permanent, and if a cure is found for HIV and AIDS within the next 10 or 15 years, you may then want to have a child. If you follow the advice about sex, you should not become pregnant, your lover should not get infected and you could still become pregnant if and when a cure is found and you have been cured.

Fatherhood

Men should not father children: you may infect the mother during sexual intercourse, or by a donation of sperm, and the mother will probably infect the child. If you have donated sperm within the last four months let the bank know that you are now infected with HIV.

Men and women

Don't donate your organs for transplantation. Keep your donor card, but write HIV across it, because otherwise someone may remember that you had a card once and not know that you have been infected.

Children

Infants born with HIV usually develop AIDS within a few months and may die within a few years. If you are the mother, you are probably infected already. The most likely cause for an older child in your family to have become infected with HIV is a blood transfusion or therapy for haemophilia (before 1985).

Children may not understand why they are ill, and different from the other children at school. They may not understand the reasons for the prejudice of their classmates and teachers against them. Only you, as a parent, can decide when to tell your child about the illness, but Chapter 12 has a list of people and organisations who understand the problems, and who can give you help and advice.

Schoolchildren get cuts and bruises more often than adults do. Teach them how to clean the cuts and bruises with antiseptic, and to cover them with waterproof dressings. Teach them how to protect their classmates and teachers from the virus in their blood. Don't let people 'kiss it better'.

If you feel able to tell the school that your child is infected, discuss with the teachers how the staff and pupils can avoid accidents, how they can improve first-aid procedures, and how they can raise the general level of hygiene in the classroom, the playground, the lavatories and the dining hall. The staff and parents are likely to appreciate your concern and help, and may accept your infected child more readily.

If you do not feel able to tell the school, discuss these things with the staff in a general way. There may be other infected children or infected teachers, about whom you don't know, and everyone will want to be safe without causing panic. Remind them that normal classroom and playground activities are quite safe, and do not transfer HIV infection. Ask the staff to discuss with you the Department of Education and Science leaflet about AIDS, and to explain how they have put it into practice.

Teenage children experiment with sex and sexual relationships. Discuss with them the nature of the sex act, and of the danger in sexual intercourse of transmitting and receiving HIV – and a large number of other venereal infections. Explain the possibility and risk of a baby being infected.

Teenagers begin to masturbate, and infected boys should know how dangerous infected semen could be to others. Teenage girls beginning to menstruate may stain their clothes and the shower rooms with infected blood. Teach them to clean spills and stains with bleach so that other children are not exposed to the virus.

Teenagers may also experiment with drugs. Try to convey the dangers of drugs and drug addiction, and the way in which drug addiction might worsen the effects of HIV infection, and might hasten the onset of AIDS. You may want to talk about tobacco addiction at the same time. You will certainly want to explain the dangers of alcohol abuse and addiction.

Teenagers often react emotionally and irrationally to parental advice. The HIV infection itself, or fear of it, may make them even more irrational. Encourage them to read this book, and as many leaflets as you can find, and persuade them to talk to someone outside the family who may have more influence than a parent.

10 Treatments for AIDS

At present there are no cures for AIDS, that is, there is no treatment that will fully restore the patient's immune response or completely remove the virus from the patient's body, but there are several ways of reducing the symptoms and of treating the opportunistic infections and some of the cancers. At the same time, many groups of doctors and scientists are working hard to find cures and vaccines.

Restoring the immune response

The opportunistic infections of AIDS take hold because the patient's immune response has been reduced or destroyed, so that restoring the response is a priority. Antibodies against the various infections (though not HIV antibodies) may be restored by infusing the patient with antibodies from other people, especially from people who have high levels. This kind of treatment has been common for cytomegalovirus infections and for shingles for some years, but unless HIV can be killed in an AIDS patient, antibody infusion is a very temporary treatment.

HIV destroys mainly the T4-lymphocytes of the immune system, but replacing these with lymphocytes from other people is not easy: they behave like transplanted organs and are rejected. Restoring the immune response of the AIDS patient is difficult and usually unsuccessful in the long term.

Treating the opportunistic infections

Control of the opportunistic infections of AIDS increases the life expectancy of the patient and improves the quality of life. However, when treatment is stopped, the underlying immune deficiency allows the same infection, or others, to recur. Antibiotics control the bacterial infections, but many of the drugs used to treat viruses, parasites and fungi have toxic side-effects, and may themselves threaten the patient's life.

The pneumonia caused by *Pneumocystis carinii*, the most common opportunistic infection, may be treated with cotrimoxazole or pentamidine, but both these drugs cause severe side-effects. Most patients experience pain at the site of injection of the drugs; some become light-headed and have abdominal pains, which may be so severe that treatment must be stopped. If this happens, or if *P. carinii* does not respond to treatment, some patients respond to a course of eflornithine hydrochloride. The side-effects of this drug are severe, and include stomach and intestinal upsets, a reversible loss of white blood cells and platelets, and, occasionally, reversible deafness.

However, candida (thrush) – one of the common infections – is easily controlled with injections of ketoconazole or amphotericin B. Similarly, the common virus infections *Herpes simplex* and *Varicella zoster* can be controlled with acyclovir, which is effective and fairly safe, even when used long term. Cytomegalovirus, another common opportunistic infection of AIDS, can be treated with ganciclovir or foscarnet, but the drugs stop the action of the virus rather than kill it and so recurrences are very frequent. Cytomegalovirus may eventually cause blindness by damaging the retina, but if treatment begins sufficiently early, a patient's sight can be saved.

Mycobacteria, which cause several forms of tuberculosis, can be treated, but not very effectively, with rifabutin, clofazimine and the new quinolones.

Some of the less frequent opportunistic infections are more difficult to treat. A number of drugs are available for toxoplasmosis (infection by organisms of the toxoplasma genus, that usually affects the brain), but their side-effects include skin allergies and loss of blood platelets. Cryptococcosis can be treated with amphotericin B, but the infection often recurs when treatment is stopped. There is currently no effective treatment for cryptosporidiosis (infection of the intestine with organisms of the cryptosporidium genus).

Treating opportunistic infections is more difficult than treating the same infections in otherwise healthy people, whose immune systems contribute toward the treatment. AIDS patients have little or no immune response, so that infections are more severe than in other people.

Anti-viral agents

There are many natural and synthetic chemicals which kill viruses, and many of them have been tested against HIV. A number of chemicals kill HIV in laboratory tests, and a few have been tested in patients. The natural chemicals include interferons, which are anti-viral chemicals produced by people who have virus infections, and interleukins, which are chemicals that stimulate lymphocytes in various ways.

The interferons have been tested extensively in the past for their activity against cancers of several kinds, and in recent years have been tested in AIDS patients. Some forms of interferon are efficient in controlling the Kaposi's sarcoma of AIDS without causing opportunistic infections. The side-effects of all forms of interferon are moderate to severe and include chills, fever, nausea, vomiting, loss of appetite, headache, loss of weight, confusion and depression. The three forms of interferon (α, β and γ) all reduce the level of virus in the blood but do not eradicate it.

Continuous infusion into patients of another of the natural chemicals, interleukin-2, has resulted in an increase in the number of lymphocytes in the blood and, in some cases, mild regression of the cancers and a reduction in the amount of virus in the blood. Another natural chemical, double-stranded ribonucleic acid, inhibits the growth of cancer cells and causes patients to make interferon. One form (now called ampligen) is not as toxic as others, and has been tested in patients. It reduces the level of virus in the patient's blood, and reduces the infectivity, in laboratory tests, of the virus, much more than does interferon.

Among the synthetic drugs, Zidovudine (which used to be called azidothymidine or AZT) stands out as being more effective than any other. The first clinical trials (held in the United States) on AIDS patients were ended early: the treated patients lived so much longer than the untreated patients that doctors decided it was unethical to withhold the drug from other patients.

Because of Zidovudine, the life expectancy of treated AIDS patients has increased. Its side-effects are severe, and include anaemia (which may mean the patient must have frequent blood transfusions), rashes, itching, nausea, headaches, confusion and convulsions. Also, it is not at all clear that the drug eradicates HIV from the body or that treatment can be stopped without a recurrence of AIDS.

Natural resistance

Healthy people who have a viral infection become immunised against the virus: they produce specific antibodies and specifically activated T-lymphocytes. This immunity neutralises the virus, and the symptoms of viral disease then disappear.

People with HIV infection produce antibodies against the virus, and a number of researchers claim that these antibodies neutralise HIV in laboratory tests, but others disagree. Very broadly, people who have a lot of neutralising antibody tend to have fewer symptoms of HIV infection. Neutralising antibodies can be detected when infected people become seropositive. In people who remain free of AIDS for some time, the level of neutralising antibody tends to increase slowly: it may be that the antibody is preventing the spread of the virus within the body. In those who develop AIDS or ARC, the amount of neutralising antibody tends gradually to fall. Neutralising antibody, when present, may also protect children infected with HIV, but the effect is neither clear-cut nor strong.

Vaccines against AIDS

A vaccine is an organism such as a virus or bacterium, or antigens (chemicals) derived from it, that has been killed or altered to prevent it causing disease. The immune system of a vaccinated person nonetheless recognises the virus or bacterium and produces antibody which will kill (or neutralise) live or unaltered virus or bacterium should it enter the body. Normally, vaccination is effective only before infection.

Several research groups and companies have attempted to prepare a vaccine effective against HIV. It may not be possible to use purified proteins or antigens from the virus, because many of the proteins from the HIV envelope are themselves immunosuppressive, and reduce the response of the immune system they are intended to stimulate. Furthermore they are relatively difficult to free completely of the live virus, and no one wants to risk injecting live virus into healthy people in order to test the vaccine.

In another form of vaccine, the genes carrying the information about the protein 'envelope' that surrounds HIV have been transfected (transferred) into a relatively harmless virus, Vaccinia. This virus normally causes cowpox, and it was used by Edward Jenner in the nineteenth century to immunise people against smallpox. The transfected virus carries an outer envelope identical to that of HIV, and so should induce immunity against HIV, and prevent infection. The value of this virus as a vaccine against HIV (and therefore against AIDS) is being studied at present. The first results suggest that the proteins in the envelope do not induce immunity, perhaps because they are immunosuppressive.

In a similar way, the envelope genes may be transferred into animal cells which are then grown in tissue culture. The cells make HIV-envelope proteins which they release into the tissue culture fluid, whence they can be purified and tested for their properties as a vaccine.

Yet another form of vaccine being tested is known as ISCOMS (for immunostimulatory complexes). Purified HIV antigens (from the virus or from cultured animal cells given HIV genes) are mixed with quill bark oil and a special detergent. Part of each HIV antigen dissolves in water and part dissolves in oil, so that the oil droplets become coated with regularly spaced HIV antigens. It is not clear whether ISCOMS will be more effective as a vaccine than transfected virus or purified antigen.

11 How do you cope with AIDS?

The first part of this chapter suggests how you might cope if you are confronted with the news that you have AIDS. The second part gives advice to others, such as family, friends and workmates of an AIDS patient.

For the patient
What the diagnosis means

From the medical point of view, the diagnosis means that your resistance to disease has been damaged by HIV, possibly beyond repair. You may have had a serious attack of pneumonia, or a virus illness, or thrush and you will probably have been admitted to hospital. It may be that you have a cancer, such as Kaposi's sarcoma. In addition you may have suffered bouts of dizziness and disorientation, perhaps felt unusually aggressive or angry. And you may have lost some control of your limbs.

On the emotional level, you may be suffering bouts of deep depression and feeling isolated from other people. Perhaps you feel angry about the way you caught the virus, and worried that your friends and family will reject you. You might also, understandably, associate your illness with sex, and the sex act may seem dangerous or frightening: because of this you and your partner may lose your desire for sex. If your partner is not infected with HIV, then intercourse will be dangerous.

The diagnosis also means that you have been to a doctor; probably one who knows a great deal about AIDS. He or she will have seen a number of other people with AIDS, and has the support of nurses, social workers, counsellors, psychologists and the Health Service.

What should you do?

You need the best medical treatment and nursing care you can find. Ask the people at the hospital or clinic for advice and help. Learn as much as you can about AIDS, its consequences and potential cures. Take part in the planning of your treatment: the medical team will welcome a positive, helpful, co-operative attitude.

In addition to medical care you should also look for emotional comfort and security. The best people to give comfort may be members of your own family and your friends, but you could also approach any of the groups listed in Chapter 12. Choose the group of people most likely to respond to your needs.

Having heard that you have AIDS, you will inevitably want to take time to think about the future. Much of the advice in Chapter 9 still holds. Consider, for example, how you want to spend your time; if you are in work and feel able to carry on, is that going to be best for you? Can you afford to give it up? Do you feel you want to investigate alternative therapies, for instance special diets and exercise regimes? Would helping other people with HIV or AIDS give you a special sense of purpose? Not everyone would feel capable of this; you shouldn't think it is necessarily expected of you. You will probably want to get your financial affairs in order, especially if you have dependents.

If possible, you should maintain your social life, or even expand it. People will notice, in time, that you are ill, but you don't have to tell them what it is if you choose not to. Try and make your daily life as stress-free as possible, in order to give your body every chance to retaliate.

What you should not do

You should not have sexual intercourse with someone who is not infected.

You should not share needles or syringes or drug-cutting equipment with people who are not infected. You should not be vaccinated (eg against polio) with 'live' virus, unless you are asked to take part in trials for an AIDS vaccine.

Most of all, for your own sake, you should not give up. Finding the will to press on may be far from easy, but you may well discover that you don't feel ill all the time. Capitalise on the good spells as much as you can, and develop a network of support that you can turn to whenever necessary.

For the carer
People with AIDS are physically ill. They may have an infectious disease, or a cancer, or both. They are often physically weak, and become weaker as time goes by. They may be thin, and they look ill.

People with AIDS are emotionally vulnerable; many are facing the prospect of death at an absurdly young age. They will almost certainly need strong emotional support and reassurance that someone cares about them, that they are worthwhile human beings.

A few people with AIDS are mentally disturbed, and are not fully in control of their movements or their behaviour. They will need special medical care.

An AIDS patient in the family, among your friends, or at work
Having someone with AIDS in the family does not mean you or anyone else will get the disease. If, however, that person is your spouse or lover, or shares needles and syringes with you, or (if you are a woman) is your own new baby, then you may already be infected with HIV. Consider being tested. You should read Chapter 9, and follow the advice we give about household hygiene.

You are most unlikely to become infected by an acquaintance, but you may want to consider who might become infected, and what you can do to prevent it, without causing panic or distress.

What can you do to help?
Perhaps the most important way of helping someone with AIDS is to provide a steady, unchanging contact with the rest of the world. An AIDS patient may become physically and mentally disoriented, and you can provide a point of contact. Where a person with AIDS might become withdrawn and isolated, you can help them to restore their social life, perhaps with a new set of friends. If they rush into an unwise course of action, you may be able to provide restraint and caution.

You can discuss the ways in which a person with AIDS can get the most enjoyment and satisfaction from life. Don't, however, expect them always to be positive; they need time to express their fears, anxieties and unhappiness.

On the practical side, you can help to contact doctors, social and welfare workers, and the self-help groups by making the first telephone calls, and perhaps by helping with transport. You could also help with the washing up, the cleaning, and in many other ways make life easier.

You may feel the person you are looking after really needs continuous professional care – which can be provided by a hospice. If you live in London you can contact the London Lighthouse or Mildmay Mission. Hospital.

Mildmay Mission Hospital (see page 119 for the address) is a charitable Christian organisation which has set up a hospice unit exclusively for the care of people with AIDS, the first in Europe. The unit contains nine individual rooms, communal relaxation areas, a counselling and support service and a home care back-up service.

The London Lighthouse (see page 132 for the address) currently provides AIDS and HIV counselling and information, buddying, crisis intervention, training in counselling and holistic health programmes. It also runs a home support service giving people with AIDS the help they need to stay in their own homes among friends and family. By the time you read this, London Lighthouse hopes to have opened a fully operational AIDS hospice, providing 24 beds for men, women or children with AIDS.

People with AIDS will also be able to get help from the Lighthouse with housing and rehousing. If members of home support teams, clinics or other AIDS organisations believe home support is not adequate, they will refer people to the hospice itself.

Remember that people who are confronting a terminal illness are often angry or depressed, and you may bear the brunt of their anger or depression, simply because you are nearest. Try to understand, to listen, and to share.

' . . . I'm not here to sit and look sick. You are only a victim if you choose to be, and I chose not to be. I'm not suffering from AIDS – I'm challenging it . . . I want to give people hope . . . that there is life after AIDS.'

'I can't say that AIDS is the best thing that ever happened to me, but it gave me a challenge, a purpose, a meaning for my life. Because suddenly it could be taken away.'

---

12 *Sources of help*

In this chapter we give details of organisations you can contact about AIDS. We start with the main AIDS charities, then go on to bodies dealing with specific groups of people (such as homosexuals, haemophiliacs and drug users), then list those concerned with specific subjects (such as employment, education and sport), and finally we list telephone helplines – both national and local. Of course, many organisations could be put under several headings, but we have listed each one under the main area it deals with. Look in the index if you can't find a particular address.

The information is as up to date as possible. We wrote to all the organisations listed asking them to fill in a questionnaire. We found that addresses and contact times can vary – particularly those of local groups. During our research several groups closed down and others were set up to take their place. For this reason you may find, for example, that you cannot get through on a certain telephone number. Don't be disheartened if this happens to you – contact a national group for advice.

We do not recommend groups or put them in any order of preference. We aim to provide sufficient information for you to turn immediately to an alternative source if necessary.

1 AIDS CHARITIES

The Terrence Higgins Trust, BM AIDS, London WC1N 3XX

Telephone   01–833 2971   Mon–Fri   7–10pm
                                          Sat–Sun   3–10pm

Telephone helpline   01–242 1010 Mon–Sun 3–10pm
Answering machine outside these hours

ADVICE   This was the first AIDS helpline in the country, set up in February 1984. General and specialist advice is given on all AIDS-related issues for everyone, straight or gay, including HIV, drugs, employment, housing, welfare benefits, health education and legal, medical and scientific topics.
ENQUIRIES   Answered by letter, telephone and appointment. Face-to-face counselling and support groups are organised for people with HIV or AIDS, their lovers, friends and family. There is also a special group for women. The Buddy Scheme is run by trained volunteers who visit people with AIDS, do chores, offer support and befriend them in general. Accommodation for those with AIDS or HIV can be arranged with housing agencies around London. The Antibody Positive Group meets in West London and links up with Body Positive – a similar independent group (see below).
LEAFLETS   *An introduction to the Trust; AIDS – the facts; AIDS and HIV; AIDS – more facts for gay men; AIDS – the straight facts (for heterosexuals); Women and AIDS; Facts about AIDS for drug users; Is it safe? The chalice and AIDS; Positive living (for HIV+ve people); AIDS and HTLV III – medical briefing; Guidelines for the provision of social and welfare services; The Trust – a newsletter; A deed of covenant to the Terrence Higgins Trust.*

Body Positive Group, PO Box 493, West Kensington, London WI4 0TF

People who are themselves HIV-positive operate a daily rota every evening (7–10pm). To find out which number to call, ring

01–242 1010	(Terrence Higgins Trust 3–10pm)
or 01–837 7324	(London Lesbian and Gay Switchboard 24 hours daily – Freefone)
or 01–359 7371	(London Friend, daily 7.30–10pm)
or (0800) 567123	(National Advisory Service on AIDS 10am–10pm Freefone)

Many regional groups offer their own support lines.

ADVICE   General and specialist advice for those who are HIV-positive, and their friends, partners and relatives. Body Positive is concerned to mobilise the individual's own resources.
ENQUIRIES   Answered by telephone, face-to-face counselling, and letter. They also run public meetings, support groups and training courses.
LEAFLETS   A fortnightly newsletter published in London.

Frontliners

ADVICE   Members all have AIDS and work together on projects producing leaflets and talking to other people with AIDS.

ENQUIRIES   Can be contacted via the Terrence Higgins Trust.

The Ibis Trust, PO Box 4QT, London W1A 4QT

Telephone   01–835 1180 (not a helpline) Mon–Sun 24 hours a day

ADVICE   General aims are to help relatives of AIDS victims, to educate people about AIDS and to help stem the spread of AIDS.
ENQUIRIES   Answered by telephone, appointment and leaflets.
LEAFLETS   *You and the HIV antibody test; Please do not open unless . . . you are interested in helping to control AIDS.*

Mildmay Mission Hospital, Hackney Road, London E2 7NA

Telephone   01–739 2331

ADVICE   An independent Christian charitable hospital serving the East End of London with an AIDS hospice unit – the first to set up in the UK. It provides individual rooms, counselling and home care.

2   GAYS AND LESBIANS

London Lesbian and Gay Switchboard, BM Switchboard, London WC1N 3XX

Telephone   01–837 7324 Mon–Sun 24 hours a day

ADVICE   A service for and staffed by gay men and women providing basic information on local gay support groups.
ENQUIRIES   Answered by telephone, sometimes by letter.

Gay Bereavement Project

ADVICE   Provides counselling and support to men or women whose partners have died, particularly just after the death. Full support in London but only telephone support in the rest of the UK.
ENQUIRIES   Can be contacted via the London Lesbian and Gay Switchboard.

3   DRUGS

SCODA (Standing Conference on Drug Abuse), 1–4 Hatton Place, Hatton Garden, London EC1N 8ND

Telephone   01–430 2341
or dial 100 and ask for 'drug problems' – this Freefone recorded message lists drug services and their telephone numbers.

ADVICE   Mostly specialist information on HIV and AIDS for drug users, but SCODA can assist with related general questions concerning employment and

119

women, for example. 'Positively women' is a self-help group for women with HIV, ARC or AIDS which meets fortnightly in the SCODA building.
ENQUIRIES   Answered by letter, leaflets and telephone.
LEAFLETS   A two-monthly newsletter; *AIDS – how drug users can avoid it; Facts about AIDS for drug workers.*

The Libra Project, Oxfordshire Council on Alcohol and Drug Use, 1 Tidmarsh Lane, Oxford OX1 1NG

Telephone   (0865) 244447 Mon–Fri 10am–5pm
Answering machine outside these hours

ADVICE   Information and counselling for alcohol and drug misusers, families and friends.
ENQUIRIES   Answered by telephone and letter; appointments can be made between 3 and 5pm; practical help is also offered. Enquirers may be referred on to organisations such as Alcoholics Anonymous, Narcotics Anonymous and Family Anon, or sometimes to alcoholic clinics.

4   BLOOD

National Blood Transfusion Service
Look in your telephone directory for details of the transfusion service nearest to you.

ADVICE   Information on people at risk who should not give blood, and for anyone worried about AIDS and considering becoming a blood donor. If you are worried that you may have contracted AIDS by blood transfusion, you should contact your doctor or the hospital where you received the transfusion – not the Blood Transfusion Service.
LEAFLET   *AIDS – what you must know before you give blood.*

The Haemophilia Society, 123 Westminster Bridge Road, London SE1 7HR

Telephone   01–928 2020
Answering machine out of office hours

ADVICE   For people with haemophilia, their friends, partners and families.
ENQUIRIES   Answered by leaflets, letter, telephone and appointments.
LEAFLETS   *What is the AIDS problem?; Haemofact* (issues connected with HIV and AIDS); *AIDS and compensation; AIDS* (presentation to The Haemophilia Society annual meeting).

Oxford Haemophilia Centre, Churchill Hospital, Headington, Oxford OX3 7LJ

Telephone   (0865) 64841 Mon–Fri 9am–5pm (not a helpline)

ADVICE Specialist advice to haemophiliacs, their families and partners.
ENQUIRIES Appointments and home visits.

5 CLINICS

To contact STD (Sexually Transmitted Disease) clinics, special clinics, GUM (genito-urinary medicine) clinics – look in the *Yellow Pages* under clinics, venereal diseases, or in the business section of your local telephone directory under venereal disease. STD clinics are often found in hospitals: they offer medical advice, counselling and testing facilities. Telephone first to find out if they offer a walk-in service or whether you need to make an appointment.

There are a number of **private clinics** – you may find one near you advertised in the telephone directory, in your local newspaper, or on stickers.

6 WOMEN AND FAMILIES

Family Planning Information Service

Telephone   01–636 7866   Mon–Thur 9am–5pm
                                            Fri 9am–4.30pm

North Thames,
FPA, 27 St Peter's Street, Bedford MK40 2PN
Telephone   (0234) 62436

South-East England
FPA, 13A Western Road, Hove BN3 1AE
Telephone   (0273) 774075

South-West England
FPA, 4 Barnfield Hill, Exeter EX1 1SR
Telephone   (0392) 56711

Wales
FPA, 6 Windsor Place, Cardiff CF1 3BX
Telephone   (0222) 42766

Eastern England
FPA, 20A Bridewell Alley, Norwich NR2 1SY
Telephone   (0603) 628704

Midlands
FPA, 5 York Road, Birmingham B16 9HX
Telephone   021–454 8236

North-West England
FPA, 104 Bold Street, Liverpool L1 4HY
Telephone   051–709 1938

Yorkshire and North-East
FPA, 17 North Church Street, Sheffield S1 2DH
Telephone   (0742) 21191

Scotland
FPA, 4 Clifton Street, Glasgow G3 7LA
Telephone   041–333 9696

London
FPA, 160 Shepherd's Bush Road, London W6 7PB
Telephone   01–602 2723

Northern Ireland
FPA, 113 University Street, Belfast BT7 1HP
Telephone   (0232) 225488

ADVICE   Well informed on questions about safer sex and the correct use of the condom, and equipped with complete lists of addresses and telephone numbers for your nearest Sexually Transmitted Disease clinic.
ENQUIRIES   Answered by letter and telephone.

Women's Reproductive Rights Information Centre (WRRIC)
52–54 Featherstone Street, London EC1Y 8RT

Telephone   01–251 6332   Office open Mon–Fri 10am–6pm (telephone first for an appointment).

ADVICE   Advice and facts on AIDS for women; detailed information on artificial insemination.
LEAFLET   *Women and AIDS.*

7   EDUCATION

Department of Education & Science (AIDS Unit), Publications Despatch Centre, Canons Park, HA7 1AZ

Telephone   01–934 9234

ADVICE   Guidance on government policy on AIDS, education about AIDS, safety and hygiene aspects in educational establishments, care of HIV-positive pupils, students and staff.
ENQUIRIES   Answered by letter.
LEAFLETS   *AIDS – some questions and answers; Children at school and problems related to AIDS.* The DES has also produced a video resource package on AIDS for use with older secondary school pupils.

Thames Television,
'Help Programme', 149 Tottenham Court Road, London W1 9LL

Telephone   01–387 9494

LEAFLETS   AIDS fact sheets plus *There are only two ways you can get AIDS* . . . and *Caring for people with HIV infection*, which are being translated into Hindi, Pumjabi, Urdu, Gujarati and Bengali. The programme has also produced a teacher's manual on AIDS, and brought out posters in association with the Health Education Authority.

The Department of Health and Social Security (Aids Unit),
Alexander Fleming House, Elephant and Castle, London SE1 6BY

Telephone   01–403 1893

Information on AIDS for doctors, dentists, teachers and local authority staff. Leaflets can be obtained direct from the DHSS Store (Health Publications Unit), PO Box 21, Stanmore, Middlesex HA7 1AY.

LEAFLETS   **AIDS – don't die of ignorance**; also various leaflets for doctors, surgeons, anaesthetists, dentists and their teams on general information and more specific topics such as artificial insemination and skin piercing.

AVERT (AIDS Virus Education and Research Trust), PO Box 91, Horsham, RH13 7YR

Telephone   (0403) 864010

ADVICE   General advice on HIV infection and AIDS; AVERT also promotes AIDS education and funding research work.
ENQUIRIES   Answered by letter, telephone and leaflets.
LEAFLETS   *Information about AIDS (updated monthly, £1); AIDS – the facts; AIDS is everyone's problem; AIDS concerns you.*

The National Union of Students, Nelson Mandela House, 461 Holloway Road, London N7 6LJ

Telephone   01–272 8900

General AIDS information for students and useful names and addresses.
LEAFLETS   *AIDS – the facts* (produced in association with AVERT); also a campaign pack for students' unions.

Guild Sound and Vision, 6 Royce Road, Peterborough PE1 5YB

Telephone   (0733) 315315

VIDEOS on AIDS for hire or purchase:

123

AIDS and you; AIDS – everyone's problem; AIDS – facts over fears; AIDS help; Coming soon.

8 MEDICAL

The Scottish Health Education Group, Woodburn House, Canaan Lane, Edinburgh EH10 4SG

Telephone   031–447 8044 (not a helpline)

ADVICE   To the general public, professional and voluntary workers.
ENQUIRIES   Answered by leaflets.
LEAFLETS   *The AIDS problem in Scotland; AIDS and sex.*

The Gay Medical Association (UK), BM/GMA, London WC1N 3XX

No telephone helpline.

ADVICE   A professional, political and social association for gay and lesbian health care professionals giving advice only to health care professionals and members of the Association. Based in London with some regional groups.
ENQUIRIES   Answered by information sheets and letter.

The Royal College of Nursing, RCN Publications Department, 20 Cavendish Square, London W1M 0AB

Telephone   01–409 3333
ADVICE   AIDS information for nursing staff.
ENQUIRIES   Answered by letter.
LEAFLETS   *AIDS – nursing guidelines.*

The Health Education Authority, 78 New Oxford Street, London WC1A 1AH

Telephone   01–631 0930 (not a helpline)

ADVICE   Gives no specialist advice or counselling, but suggests other organisations.
ENQUIRIES   Answered by leaflets and referrals, for instance to the AIDS Information Service and the National Advisory Service.
LEAFLETS   *Learning about AIDS – what everybody needs to know; AIDS in schools; AIDS and professionals; Some facts about AIDS;* also a resources centre for schools.

North-West Thames Regional Health Authority, 40 Eastbourne Terrace, London W2 3QR

Telephone   01–262 8011 (ext 3252 – not a helpline)

They supply the St Mary's Pack to District Health Authorities containing information on such topics as disinfection, serum storage and domestic services.

British Medical Association, BMA House, Tavistock Square, London WC1H 9JP

Telephone   01–387 4499

LEAFLET   (In co-operation with the BBC AIDS campaign) *AIDS – the positive approach (£1).*

9   EMPLOYMENT

The Health and Safety Executive (HSE), Library and Information Services, Baynards House, 1 Chepstow Place, Westbourne Grove, London W2 4TF

Telephone 01–221 0870 Mon–Fri 10am–3pm

The Health and Safety Executive HSE), Library and Information Services, Broad Lane, Sheffield S3 7HQ

Telephone   (0742) 752539

The Health and Safety Executive (HSE), Library and Information Services, St Hugh's House, Stanley Precinct, Bootle, Merseyside L20 3QY

Telephone   051–951 4381

ADVICE   Details on the health, safety and welfare of people at work and the public who may be affected in that connection. Specific information on AIDS for health service employees.
ENQUIRIES   Answered by telephone, letter and leaflets.
LEAFLETS   *AIDS and employment; AIDS – prevention of infection in the health services; Revised guidelines on AIDS* (produced by the Advisory Committee on Dangerous Pathogens); the HSE also keep a catalogue of medical and hygiene subject matters.

Employment Medical Advisory Services (EMAS)
Part of the HSE, this is a national network of doctors and nurses which gives free advice about AIDS – and other occupational health matters – to employers, employees and trade unions. Addresses and telephone numbers can be found in the business sections of local directories under **Health and Safety Executive.**

Department of Employment, Information division, Caxton House, Tothill Street, London SW1H 9NF

Telephone   01–213 3000 (not a helpline)

ADVICE   Guidance for employers on AIDS, levels of risk, rights and procedures.
LEAFLETS   *AIDS and employment.*

COHSE, (Confederation of Health Service Employees),
Glen House, High Street, Banstead, Surrey SM7 2LH

Telephone   (073 73) 53322

ADVICE   Information on AIDS specifically for health service employees.
ENQUIRIES   Answered by letter, telephone, leaflets and appointments.
LEAFLETS   *Health and safety bulletin – guidelines for health staff; Hepatitis B – guidelines for health staff.*

10   COUNSELLING

National Association of Citizens Advice Bureaux,
115–123 Pentonville Road,
London N1 9LZ

Telephone   01–833 2181

ADVICE   Only to other Citizens Advice Bureaux, not to the public. Addresses and telephone numbers of all local bureaux can be found in the business sections of local telephone directories.

British Association for Counselling, 37a Sheep Street, Rugby, Warwickshire CV21 3BX

Telephone   (0788) 78328

ADVICE   Supplies names of local counsellors and counselling agencies and information on training in counselling those with AIDS.
LEAFLET   *Counselling and AIDS* (a list of useful contacts and addresses).

Office of the Chief Rabbi, *(Sir Immanuel Jakobovits),* Adler House, Tavistock Square, London WC1H 9HN
LEAFLET   *AIDS – Jewish perspectives.*

11   SPORTS ASSOCIATIONS

The Rugby Football Union, Twickenham TW1 1DZ

Telephone   01–892 8161 (not a helpline)

ENQUIRIES   Answered by letter, telephone and appointments.
LEAFLET   *The hazards of AIDS and injury.*

The Sports Council, 16 Upper Woburn Place, London WC1H 0QP

Telephone   01–388 1277

ENQUIRIES   Answered by press cuttings about AIDS and sports.
LEAFLET   *AIDS and swimming pools.*

12   TELEPHONE INFORMATION

Healthline (College of Health)

Telephone   01–980 4848   Mon–Sun 2–10pm

ADVICE   Operators will play one of the following tapes selected by the caller.

No 228   Guide to the College of Health AIDS Information Service
No 136   What is AIDS?
No 229   Who is at risk of contracting AIDS? – the main groups
No 230   Testing for AIDS: what test is available, what it shows and where you can have it done
No 231   AIDS: information for young people
No 232   Symptoms and signs of AIDS
No 233   AIDS and women
No 234   Safer sex for heterosexuals worried about AIDS
No 235   Safer sex for gay men and bisexuals
No 236   Safer sex for haemophiliacs worried about AIDS
No 237   Safer sex for drug users worried about AIDS
No 238   AIDS and the workplace
No 239   AIDS and blood transfusions
No 240   AIDS and artificial insemination
No 241   How you can help someone who has AIDS.
No 242   What to do if you are HIV positive

Four other services are similar to the London Healthline but give local information about clinics and organisations you might like to contact.

Exeter (0392) 59191
Basingstoke (0256) 471438
Hull (0482) 29933
Croydon 01–681 3311

Healthline also operates a 24-hour automatic information service: tapes are played direct to the caller without the need to go through an operator.

General information and useful names and addresses:

01–981 2717 (local rates from London)
01–980 7222 (local rates from London)
(0345) 581151 (local rates outside London)

Safer sex for heterosexuals:

01–981 7112 (local rates from London)
(0345) 581876 (local rates outside London)
(0800) 010976 (free from anywhere in the UK)

Safer sex for gay men and bisexuals:
  01–981 7188 (local rates from London)
  (0345) 581881 (local rates outside London)
  (0800) 010981 (free from anywhere in the UK)
AIDS and young people:
  01–981 7140 (local rates from London)
  (0345) 581858 (local rates outside London)
  (0800) 010958 (free from anywhere in the UK)

LEAFLETS *Healthline Directory; AIDS – beyond the adverts; AIDS and the government.*

Department of Health and Social Security AIDS Information Service and the National Advisory Service

Telephone   (0800) 555777 (free)

This is the number printed on the government's AIDS leaflet dropped into every household in the UK at the beginning of 1987. If you phone the number and give your address you will be sent a detailed booklet about AIDS.

National Advisory Service on AIDS

Telephone   (0800) 567123 (free)
Phone this number between 10 in the morning and 10 at night to get direct answers from a trained adviser to your questions about AIDS.

A conmmercially run information line consisting of four-minute long tapes on various aspects of AIDS:

AIDS (general)	(0898) 600699
AIDS and drug users	(0898) 600900
Facts and news	(0898) 600901
AIDS and men	(0898) 600902
Schoolchildren	(0898) 600903
Sex	(0898) 600904
Sport	(0898) 600905
Tests and transfusions	(0898) 600906
Women and pregnancy	(0898) 600907
AIDS in the workplace	(0898) 600908

All (0898) numbers are charged at 25p a minute during standard and cheap times, and at 38p a minute during peak time.

People who are hard of hearing with access to Vistel machines can ring (0800) 521361 to get general information on AIDS.

Anyone needing information on AIDS in Hindi, Punjabi, Gujarati, Bengali, Urdu or Cantonese can ring 01–992 5522.

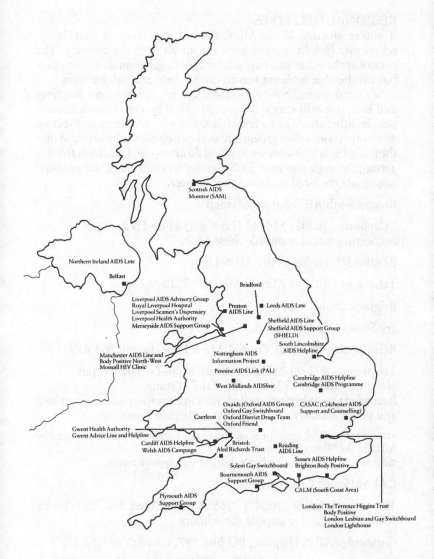

AIDS helplines and support groups.

REGIONAL HELPLINES

If you're worried about AIDS, the quickest route to help is the telephone. Helplines have been set up all over the country. The person at the other end may not be able to give you all the answers but will be able to direct you to further help and information.

We must stress, however, that these are independent helplines and each one will vary – some are backed by very knowledgeable people, others have just a few volunteers who are better at directing you to specialists than giving advice themselves. We have found that the times the telephones are manned do alter – so if you have trouble getting through you may find it easier to call one of the national organisations listed earlier in this chapter.

Bournmouth AIDS Support Group

Telephone   (0202) 424442 (Freefone) Mon–Fri 8–10pm
Answering machine outside these hours

Bradford/West Yorkshire AIDS Line

Telephone   (0274) 732939 Mon–Fri 7.30–9.30pm

Brighton Body Positive

See Sussex AIDS Helpline.

Bristol: Aled Richards Trust, 1 Mark Lane, Bristol BS1 4XR

Telephone   (0272) 297963 (office) Mon–Fri 10am–4pm
Helpline   (0272) 273436 Mon–Fri 7–11pm
Recorded tape when not staffed, with information on opening times and phone number of The Terrence Higgins Trust.

ADVICE   Practical, emotional and financial support to anyone affected by AIDS in the West of England.
ENQUIRIES   Answered by letter, leaflets and appointments.

CALM (South Coast Area)

Telephone helpline   (0243) 776998 Mon, Wed, Fri 7.30–10pm
Answering machine outside these hours

Cambridge AIDS Helpline, PO Box 257, Cambridge CB2 1XQ

Telephone   (0223) 69765 Tue, Wed 7.30–10pm
Trained volunteers provide a buddy service for people with AIDS, face-to-face counselling, Body Positive self-help group, liaison with drugs project in Cambridge.

Cambridge AIDS Programme, AIDS Education Unit, Foxton House, Adrian Way, Long Road, Cambridge CB2 2SQ

Telephone   (0223) 410458/245151
This organisation coordinates all AIDS-related activities in the Cambridge Health Authority area.

LEAFLET   *Worried about AIDS?*

Cardiff AIDS Helpline

Telephone   (0222) 40101 Mon–Fri 7–10pm

ADVICE   General and specialist advice covering all AIDS-related subjects.
ENQUIRIES   Answered by telephone, letter and face-to-face counselling. (Their line is shared with the Welsh AIDS Campaign.)

CASAC (Colchester AIDS Support and Counselling)
(Essex, Suffolk & Norfolk areas)

Telephone helpline   (0206) 42980 Tue, Fri 7.30–10pm
Answering machine outside these hours

Gwent Health Authority, Mill Street, Caerleon, Gwent NP6 1XG

Telephone Advice line   (0633) 422532 Tue 2–8pm
                Helpline   (0633) 841901 Mon–Fri 8.30am–4.30pm
                (except Thur pm)

ADVICE   These are independent lines financed by the Health Authority and run by trained AIDS counsellors. Advice is given on all AIDS-related issues except finance and insurance.
LEAFLETS   *AIDS – a serious concern for all of us; AIDS – what it means for young people; Recommendations for professionals who may come into contact with people with AIDS.* The Health Authority also lends out within Gwent a teaching pack about AIDS.

Leeds AIDS Line

Telephone helpline   (0532) 444209 Mon, Wed, Thur Fri 7–9pm
Answering machine outside these hours

Liverpool AIDS Advisory Group, St Peter's Church, Church Avenue, Liverpool L9 4SG

Telephone   051–521 8819 or 526 6118 Mon–Fri 10am–10pm,
                Sat 10am–12 noon

Information and advice on HIV testing:

Royal Liverpool Hospital, Prescot Street, Liverpool L7 8XN

Telephone   051–709 0141

Seamen's Dispensary, Cleveland Buildings, Liverpool L1 5BH

Telephone   051–709 2165 For men only

Talks and training workshops:
Liverpool Health Authority,
Health Education Officer – AIDS, Sefton General Hospital, Smithdown Road, Liverpool L15 2HE

Telephone   051–733 4020

London – *see also:*
The Terrence Higgins Trust, Body Positive and the London Lesbian and Gay Switchboard (all at the beginning of this chapter).

London Lighthouse, 178 Lancaster Road, London W11 1QU

Telephone   01–221 6513 and 01–727 2018 (due to change mid-1988)

ADVICE   Counselling and advice for people who have AIDS or are HIV-positive.

Manchester AIDS Line and Body Positive North-West,
PO Box 201, Manchester M60 1PU

Telephone   061–228 1617 Mon–Fri 7–10pm

Body Positive (Manchester)

Telephone   061–228 2212 Tue, Thur 7–10pm
Recorded tape outside office hours

Merseyside AIDS Support Group,
PO Box No 11, Liverpool L69 1SN
Telephone   051–709 9000 (office)
Telephone helpline   051–709 9000 Mon, Wed, Fri 7–10pm

ADVICE   General and specialist, home service volunteer scheme. The Body Positive group meets weekly on Tuesdays.
ENQUIRIES   Answered by telephone, leaflets and letter.
LEAFLETS   *Fashionable to think about AIDS; Drug injectors and AIDS; AIDS and the condom; Avoiding AIDS.* They also supply material from the Liverpool Drug Information Centre, for instance.
See also Liverpool AIDS Advisory Group.

Monsall HIV Clinic, Monsall Road, Newton Heath,
Manchester M10 8WR

Telephone   061–205 2393

ADVICE   General and specialist, although insurance and benefit claims are referred elsewhere.
ENQUIRIES   Answered by telephone, appointments, counselling and leaflets.
LEAFLETS   *Play safely; AIDS – what every woman needs to know; What about AIDS testing?*

Northern Ireland AIDS Line, PO Box 206, Belfast BT1 1SJ

Telephone   (0232) 326117 Mon, Fri 7.30–10pm
Answering machine outside these hours

ADVICE   General on all aspects of HIV infection, backed up by other organisations' leaflets.
ENQUIRIES   Personal meetings arranged if necessary.

Nottingham AIDS Information Project,
c/o CUS, 33 Mansfield Road, Nottingham NG1 3FF

Telephone helpline (0602) 585526 Mon, Tue, Wed 7–10pm and various times during the day.
Answering machine outside these hours

Nottingham AIDS Information Project,
c/o The Self-Help Team, 114 Mansfield Road,
Nottingham NG1 3HL

ADVICE   General advice on all AIDS-related issues. Buddy training courses and a self-help team.
ENQUIRIES   Answered by leaflets, talks, telephone and letter.
LEAFLETS   *Safer sex – a guide for gay men; AIDS and women; AIDS and you; AIDS – a concern for all; AIDS and prostitution.*

Oxaids (Oxford AIDS Group), Harrison Department,
Genito-urinary medicine, Radcliffe Infirmary, Woodstock Road,
Oxford OX2 6HE

Telephone   (0865) 728817 Sun, Mon, Wed 6–8pm
                                  Fri 2–4pm
Answering machine outside these hours

ADVICE   General.
ENQUIRIES   Answered by telephone and appointment.
On the same number, the GU (Genito-urinary) Clinic gives general

information to anyone who asks. They also hold a walk-in clinic (Mon–Fri 1–3pm) for those anxious about HIV.

Oxford Gay Switchboard

Telephone   (0865) 726893 Mon, Thur, Sat, Sun 7–9pm

ADVICE   Specialist AIDS advice for gay men and women on health.
ENQUIRIES   Answered by telephone and appointment.

Oxford District Drugs Team, Ley Clinic, Littlemore Hospital, Oxford OX4 4XN

Telephone   (0865) 718440 (ext 70) Mon–Fri 9am–5pm
Answering machine outside these hours

ADVICE   Advice on HIV particularly for drug users.
ENQUIRIES   Answered by letter, telephone, leaflets and appointments.

Oxford Friend, c/o 34 Cowley Road, Oxford OX4 1HZ

Telephone   (0865) 726893 Tue, Wed, Fri 7–9pm

ADVICE   General and specialist AIDS advice for gay people.
ENQUIRIES   Answered chiefly by telephone, but also by letter and appointments.
LEAFLET   *Oxford friend – helps gay people.*

Pennine AIDS Link (PAL), PO Box 167, Bradford, West Yorkshire BD1 1LL

Telephone   (0274) 732939 helpline
Mon–Fri 7.30–9.30pm (usually)
Answering machine outside these hours

ADVICE   On all AIDS-related issues, particularly the HIV test. PAL serves the Pennines side of West Yorkshire and is setting up a training programme for volunteer face-to-face counselling and buddying.
ENQUIRIES   Answered mainly by telephone.
LEAFLETS   From The Terrence Higgins Trust, the Health Education Council and the local Health Promotion Unit.

Plymouth AIDS Support Group, Special Clinic, Freedom Fields Hospital, Plymouth

Telephone   (0752) 229817 (not a helpline)

ADVICE   General support, specialist counselling in association with local health advisers.
ENQUIRIES   When you ring, the Clinic will put you in touch with a member of the Support Group.

Preston AIDS Line

Telephone   (0772) 555556 helpline,
Mon, Tue, Thur 7.30–9.30pm
Answering machine outside these hours

Reading AIDS Line, AIDS Support Group, PO Box 358, Reading RG6 3GD

Telephone   (0734) 503377 Mon, Thur 8–10pm

ADVICE   By telephone and letter.

Scottish AIDS Monitor (SAM), PO Box 169, Edinburgh EH1 3UU

Telephone helplines:
    Edinburgh 031–558 1167 Mon–Sun 7.30–10pm
    Glasgow   041–221 7467 Tue–Thur 7–10pm
    Dundee   (0382) 200532 Tue–Thur 7–10pm
    Aberdeen   (0224) 574000 Tue, Fri   7–10pm
Answering machine outside these hours

ADVICE   On all aspects of AIDS and HIV infection. They hold an annual conference and occasional seminars.
ENQUIRIES   See above for helpline numbers. They also answer letters.
LEAFLETS   *Advice and information for drug users and sexual partners; SAM speaks; Living gay – loving safe; Women and AIDS; AIDS and teenagers.*

Sheffield AIDS Line

Telephone   (0742) 755500 Mon, Thur 7–10pm

ADVICE   Counselling by phone. Plans for training courses for volunteer counsellors. Affiliated to the Sheffield AIDS Support Group (SHIELD) which runs a buddying training scheme.

Solent Gay Switchboard

Telephone   (0703) 37363 Tue, Thur, Sat 7.30–10pm

ADVICE   Counselling by phone for gay men and women.

South Lincolnshire AIDS Helpline

Telephone:
    (0476) 60192 Mon, Fri 9–10am, Wed 1–3pm
    (0205) 54462 Mon 12 noon–2pm, Thur 3.30–5.30pm
Answering machine outside these hours

ADVICE   General and specialist.

ENQUIRIES   Followed up by trained AIDS counsellors.
LEAFLET   *Special diseases and conditions – acquired immune deficiency syndrome.*

Sussex AIDS Helpline/Brighton Body Positive, PO Box 17, Brighton BN2 5NQ

Telephone   (0273) 571660   Mon–Sun 8–10pm

ADVICE   General and specialist – experts available on HIV, women and gays. Counselling and care group; women's group; buddy scheme.
ENQUIRIES   Answered by letter, telephone, and leaflets.
LEAFLETS   *Get the facts; HIV antibody positive; Women and AIDS; Safer sex.*

Welsh AIDS Campaign, PO Box 348, Cardiff CF1 4XL

Telephone   (0222) 40101   Mon–Fri office hours and 7–10pm (shared with Cardiff AIDS helpline)

ADVICE   Primarily coordinates and devises education and prevention strategies throughout Wales.
ENQUIRIES   Answered by telephone and letter.

West Midlands Aids Line, 4th Floor, Smithfield House, Digbeth, Birmingham B5 6BS

Telephone helpline   021–622 1511   Mon–Fri 7.30–10pm

ADVICE   General and specialist advice on all HIV- and AIDS-related issues, including safer sex, healthier lifestyles and insurance.
ENQUIRIES   Answered by leaflets, letter, telephone and face-to-face counselling.

Index

Key words, such as body fluids, haemophilia – and, of course, HIV and AIDS themselves – appear throughout the book as well as on the pages indicated.